Joyce,

Why Can't I Lose Weight?
TOXINS

Curing 18 Diseases My Doctors Couldn't With A 35 Pound Weight
Loss! Learn About Hormones, Adrenals, Infections,
Toxic Fat and Toxic Teeth.

Cheers!
To Great Health
and Happiness.
Lisa

LISA HEATHER TORBERT

ISBN: 1503276031
ISBN 13: 9781503276031
Cover Artist : Aekyung Maria Ruffin
Author Photo by: David Wolanski

TABLE OF CONTENTS

To My Family................

I would like to take this opportunity to shine a spotlight of admiration on my husband Mark. I would like to honor him by expressing my sincere appreciation for the time he dedicated to reading and proofing this book. Most of you will not understand how big a job this book was for Mark, not only having to clean up the mess in my book, but going without dinners, the endless clutter I no longer had time to deal with and putting up with my head in the book for ten hours a day. My husband is someone who always has my back, my confidant who supports all my crazy ventures........ my rock! I am the luckiest women in the world to have someone that I can just kick back with, laugh with, or scream with at a rock concert. So thank you Mark for supporting my dreams, for supporting me and most of all for being the luckiest man in the world to have me! I love the hell out of you.

I would like to dedicate this book to my husband and our beautiful; five children, their spouse, our six grandchildren and our parents. Here's to all of the wonderful times we have shared together and to the special times we look forward to. There is no greater love that we share, than the special love between family and friends. It's more than love, It's the fun and laughter we have, the bonds we make, the closeness we share whether healing a tragedy or enjoying a celebration.

Sometimes I am the teacher.....

      Sometimes the student and

         Sometimes the lesson

I love you all..... even when we are messy.

1

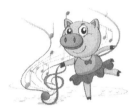

"DOUBLE YOUR PLEASURE, DOUBLE YOUR BUN"
WHY AM I FAT?

"Just a Spoon Full of Sugar" My Childhood

I think I was born fat. I can't really remember ever being thin. My mom used the word plump and every year we traveled an hour away from our home to buy ½ size clothes. However, the worst memories are the boys who called me names; Tank was their favorite. When I was 11 we used to play a neighborhood game where the boys chased the girls and if they caught us they would kiss us. Because of my "tootsie roll" there were no "kisses" for me. All jokes aside, the pain was more than skin deep lasting most of my lifetime. I remember staring into the mirror, always looking with disapproval, wondering "Who's the Fattest of them all." At the age of 8, I remember sitting in front of the tube watching Hee Haw with my family. When the dancing pigs came across the screen my brother said "Hey that looks like Lisa". I ran upstairs crying and devastated.

My brother was only 6 at the time and was not trying to insult me; I was enrolled in ballet classes and wore a tutu like the pigs wore. When you are fat, all you think about is being fat. You take everything to heart. No wonder I grew up being such a freak about my weight. You can read more about emotional weight gain and perception in Chapter 16, Mirror, Mirror.

When you start young eating an unhealthy diet, most poor eating habits will continue into your adulthood and possibly for the rest of your life. I grew up in the sixties, the invention of fast food restaurants, frozen processed foods and penny candy. Can you say Burger Chef? My mom was an alcoholic and my dad worked many hours to support our family. I actually grew up like a lot of the kids are today, eating fast foods, processed foods and frozen foods. Most families in the sixties thought TV dinners were a treat. In my family we ate TV dinners often and almost always in front of the television. In addition to those unhealthy meals, I consumed lots of junk; cupcakes, cookies, candy, pretzels, pop tarts and cereal. Everything I ate was unhealthy. The penny candy store was conveniently located right down the street from my school. I stopped daily on the way home to pick up my treats. I never had many friends come over to my house since my mom was sick and usually sleeping during the day. I felt lonely at a very early age, and started down a very *"rocky road"*. I did not find *"mounds of joy"* so *my "life savers"* were dreaming I was a "tiny *tart"* instead of a *"whopper."*

At the age of 5, I was constantly ill so my parents agreed with the doctors to have my tonsils and adenoids removed. I was always on antibiotics and also had tubes put into my ears. Nothing helped, so the doctors thought I should get tested for allergies. The results showed I was allergic to milk, cats, dust, and many other allergens. My father had to drive me an hour away to my allergist to get weekly shots, until he finally administered the shots himself. Allergies were not common back then and we had no allergist in our local town. I remained on allergy shots until the age of 30.

"Bad to the Bone "My Teen Years

At the age of 13, my mom took me to my family doctor, and believe it or not, he gave me a prescription for Preludin, an amphetamine. I did not like the racy feeling, but the results were great as I finally started to lose weight. At 14, I was already a hot mess; killing off brain cells with alcohol and drugs and very low self-esteem. I started to get urinary tract infections at the age of 15 and had to have my urethra dilated many times. At age 16, I went to my dentist for my annual visit and was told I had 17 cavities. Who has this many cavities? Crazy! More about this in Chapter 11. I also had frequent visits to the hospital for abdominal pain, which turned out that my colon was impacted. I was very constipated which was a combo of stress and poor food choices.

"Nothing Taste as good as Thin" Twenties

I was still doing the amphetamines to keep my weight down. I noticed by my twenties I had developed food allergies. I was gluten intolerant and so when I ate wheat or dairy I would swell up. Then I developed Candidiasis, chronic yeast infections. I also used antibiotics for my frequent urinary tract infections a deadly cycle. I also had mono and was later diagnosed with Epstein Barr. My weight fluctuated up and down; and I'm not talkin bout a couple pounds, I was gaining 10 to 20. Gain and lose, up and down, drugs and starvation, I was a chronic yoyo dieter.

So you can catch my drift, my life of unhealthy eating and drug use was definitely affecting my health. At some point I knew it wasn't right, but that did not stop me from using the prescription weight loss drugs. I had to *use it to lose it;* and if I didn't use them I would eat and gain. Being thin was the most incredible feeling that most people take for granted. I felt acceptable, normal like my friends who were thin. I eventually got the doctor to give me a script for Hydrochlorothiazide, fluid pills and bam, I could lose five pounds in one day; the difference between fitting into my pants or not. So I was addicted early on.

The big but, (no pun intended), is that the damage was already done. Getting no nutrition in my diet for most of my life made me very sick. My unhealthy lifestyle would set me up for a lifetime of infection. Throw in two car accidents, age 13 and 16, in a time where most did not wear a seatbelt and as you can see I was on the "Highway to Hell."

To add fuel to the fire, my mom was addicted to speed and booze. I was not only physically ill, but like my mom, I was mentally and emotionally sick. I was also married and divorced twice in my twenties. The best part of my twenties was the birth of my son. It was the best choice I ever made in my life as I was dedicated to giving him a life filled with love and attention. I quit smoking while I was pregnant; I made homemade baby food, and always made sure we were surrounded with family, friends and activities. He was never sick as a child and is still a very healthy person. I did what I set out to do, make his life the opposite of mine, Healthy.

"Thirty and Rockin"

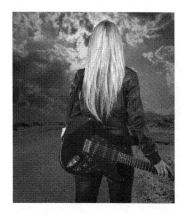

At the age of 30, I had already been performing in bands for the last ten years as a singer, guitar player and keyboardist. I was no slacker, so I carried all of the heavy equipment, just like the guys. I had to keep up my "reputation" and had to starve myself to stay as small as possible. And we know it's over "*if the fat lady sings.*" Band members did not want a fat singer! Although I was not "*rockin wellness*" yet, I did quit smoking (a 15 year old habit) and become a vegetarian.

I continued to have neck pain from my car accidents and I started going to a chiropractor who put me on the road to healing. He helped me with my food allergies and candida and recommended colon hydrotherapy, since I was constipated often and suffered from Irritable Bowel Syndrome (IBS). This was back in the day where the only colon hydrotherapy was in places like NYC and California. I purchased my own colonic board so I could start doing my own colon hydrotherapy at home. With the combination of the candida diet and colonics, I started to feel fantastic. Most of my thirties I would continue to bounce up and down with my weight. I would lose and gain the same 10 pounds over and over, but for the most part, I was able to stay fairly slim. The weird thing is I thought I was fat, when I was really very thin. I was 5'5 and weighed 130 pounds. I continued to try every diet there was; Weight Watchers, Adkins, Nutra System, Jenny Craig, LA Weight Loss, Cabbage Soup Diet, Grapefruit diet, Body for Life, Eat Right for Your Blood Type, etc. I also ordered every weird thing I saw on television that gave me hope; appetite suppressors, creams, detox wraps, stretch bands and so on. I started running and ran up to six miles four times a week for probably 5 years. This was a great help with my weight until I herniated my L5 disk in my back and had to stop running. I was feeling pretty good in my thirties, staying with my gluten free/candida diet and was able to stay thin. When I was thin, I was the happiest person on earth. It just felt *"so right to be light."*

"Forty, Life Starts Here"

Well, it did not start well for me; I was getting sicker and heavier. It was becoming harder and harder to keep my weight down. The years of my child-hood antibiotics, prescription weight loss drugs, and infected teeth all started to take their toll, although I would not figure this out for another 10 years. However, I did become an expert at fulfilling my role as the "Adult Child of an Alcoholic" by abusing my addictions of; workaholic, chronic dieting and exer-cise addiction. Thank God I had made it through my experimental teenage years, and did not enjoy consuming more than an occasional drink since my early twenties. Alcohol and drugs, just not my thing, but my work addictions took me to a whole other level and just as dangerous. Work was my favor-ite drug. Workaholics enjoy norepinephrine, a neurotransmitter that produces "chemical enjoyment." I spent my life building empires, trying to prove myself as worthy. Low self-esteem crept into all aspects of my life. I pushed myself at the gym, did a lot of construction work on rentals I had bought, and worked at least 50 – 60 hours a week. At 45, I went back to college and received my Master's Degree in Community Counseling. I worked for years helping people to recover from their addictions. My best client, ta-da, was myself; healing the old wounds that scarred my life. My emotional healing was great, but I was the heaviest weight in my life.

"Caution Middle Age Meltdown" Fifty

When I turned 50, I did have a medical meltdown, my body was burned out. My life came to an abrupt stop. I had just worked myself to the bone, well not really. At 50, I put on 50, pounds that is! I became increasing scared because I no longer had control over my weight; I was physically working out hard, eating very little, and the scales were not budging. I had just finished building my brand new holistic health center, and I was exhausted. I was not only the builder, I did a lot of construction myself, not to mention all the chemicals I was exposed to during demolition and building. After opening up my new center, I shut down! I had to stay home; I was not even able to enjoy my new accomplishment. I visited many medical doctors that would diagnose me with diabetes, heart arrhythmia and vertigo. I went to a specialist for adrenal issues and the docs told me my adrenals were fine. So why couldn't I get out of bed? I had no energy at all. Most of the docs I visited prescribed anti-depressants, which I declined. I told them I was sick not depressed. I remember leaving the doctor's office so confused. I was beyond exhaustion and my vertigo limited every normal function. My eyes were bloodshot and burning, and I had to hold on to the wall when walking. The one thing I did realize was that a lifetime of stress and pushing myself, being a workaholic, contributed to my illnesses. After about six months of researching illnesses, I finally diagnosed myself with adrenal fatigue. Most doctors do not acknowledge adrenal fatigue, so this made it really hard to heal. After a year of going from doctor to doctor, including holistic practitioners, I was not any better. I had every test conceivable and they found nothing. I felt so discouraged. I felt so misunderstood. I was harboring my fears that I was never going to get well again, let alone slim down. At this point in my life, it was impossible for me to lose weight, no matter what I did. I tried to put on a happy face, but it was all such a lie, I was "*Slipping into darkness.*"

At age 51, I found a remarkable company, Premier Research Labs, which changed my life forever. Being a holistic health practitioner allowed me to join the Premier family and become educated on their protocol. I explained my symptoms and they sent me supplements to help my conditions and taught me how to start a detox system. After a couple of weeks, I started to feel better. After a couple of months I was back to work part time. In the next six months I would heal myself from five different disorders, including all of my food allergies. This had such an impact on my life. I decided put my counseling career on the back burner and began training to become a, Quantum Reflex Analysis (QRA) Practitioner, working with Premier Research Labs. I use QRA to test people for nutritional deficiencies and disease, the process I used to heal myself. More on QRA in Chapter 13.

"Buckle Up, Difficult Life Change"

"*I Can't Drive 55*". I wanted to drive 100mph and speed right through the next couple of years. At the age of 55, I thought I had been through enough, but no, the worst was yet to come. I started failing again. My vertigo came back and I was diagnosed with fibromyalgia. I was like a cripple, especially when I had to get up and walk. In 2012 I was at my yearly Premier Research Labs training in Texas where I listened to the guest speaker, Dr. Sambatara, who was a holistic dentist in Ellicot City, MD, that actually lives two hours from my home. He informed us that he had proven studies that all root canal teeth still held infection in them. I told him I had ten root canal teeth and he said I would need to have all of those teeth and roots removed. He told me there was no way to save the teeth. I was SHOCKED! I was so sick at that point, I started getting my teeth removed. Just as Dr. Sambatara told me, all my teeth were infected. He sent a sample of my tissue from just one of my tooth removals and had it tested. The results were the proof in the pudding; 16 different infections from just one tooth, and five were listed as high risk. Read more and see my results chart in chapter 11.

Holy Molar! In addition to my extractions, and tissue removals also came mercury removals, and amalgam tattoos, where the mercury had to be cut from my gum where it was leaking out. So I became toothless, having to invest in an upper and bottom plate. After the eighth tooth was removed, so was my fibromyalgia. I have had no return of my fibromyalgia since.

With my fibromyalgia gone, I noticed that my thoracic back pain was getting worse. Unfortunately, I have a high tolerance for pain, so after four years of serious pain, I decided to have an MRI. My spinal MRI showed I had Syringomyelia. Say what? I had a syrinx, a sack filled with spinal fluid, stretching out in my spinal canal in thoracic area of my spine at T-10 and T-11. Syringomyelia is a rare spinal cord injury that enlarges over time and causes more damage and deterioration to the nerve centers of the spinal cord because of the pressure from the fluid. My syrinx was already large, an inch and three quarters in length by a half inch wide. I didn't deserve this and I was angry. I had a rare disorder which would eventually need surgery. There are only 8 in 100,000 people that are diagnosed with Syringomyelia. I was able to reduce my pain from a 10 to a 0-3 on most days with my holistic practices, mostly a mud detoxing clay that I applied daily. This bought me two years. I signed up for a study at the NIH and was accepted into the program. I was informed that many people develop a syrinx from trauma, like car accidents and from lifting. My accidents were over 40 years ago, but my life time of physical abuse had caught up with me.

The pain in my back was starting to get worse again and I was unable to reduce the pain any longer. In July of 2014, I awoke to the worst migraine headache I ever had in my life and then I was dizzy for the next 6 weeks. I scheduled my last root canal removal and like magic it disappeared immediately. Because I was dizzy, I did not notice, or maybe I was in denial, that I was having an increase in the nerve impulses running down my legs. It was also much harder to climb stairs. I called the NIH to talk with my doctor and he told me it was time for surgery. If I did not have the surgery, it would not be long before I would be in a wheelchair. Surgery went well, but I woke up numb from the waist down. I have lost the strength in my legs making it hard to climb stairs. By the time I had surgery, I knew I had waited too long, since I already experienced loss of strength and nerve impulses racing down my legs.

Currently I have regained about 50% of the sensation/feeling in my lower body and have started physical therapy. I am still optimistic that I will have a full recovery and I am thankful that I can now walk without a cane.

My healing has been an amazing journey. I have healed from 19 different diseases/disorders listed on the next page.

- Irregular Heart Beat
- Diabetes
- Vertigo
- Adrenal Fatigue
- Gluten Intolerant
- Onion Allergy
- Fibromyalgia
- Restless Leg Syndrome
- Thyroid Issues
- Depression
- Hormone Imbalance
- 10 toxic root canals
- Epstein Barr
- Irritable Bowel Syndrome
- Urinary Tract Infections
- Candida
- Lyme Disease
- Hair loss/ thinning
- 26 year old corn on toe

I have a lifetime of losses, but have gained a wealth of knowledge that I can now pass on to everyone that is sick and tired of being sick, tired and overweight. This is my personal weight loss journey. With my personal experience, I offer life changing techniques to help you lose the weight, keep it off and restore your body to a healthy state.

So here is where the real story begins for you; a complete book on how to detox and lose weight.

Why Can't I Lose Weight? Toxins!

2

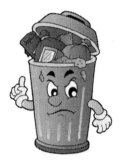

"ROTTEN TO THE CORE" TAKING OUT THE GARBAGE

I think the first week is definitely the hardest, getting rid of the stinkiest garbage in our diets. I am not going to "*sugar coat it*", so this is not only the most important part of your journey, but it will be a constant challenge.

Fast Foods

Our first stop is the drive through window at some of our favorite restaurants, *"Home of the Whopper, It's Good Mood Food,"* and *"Finger Lickin' Good"*. These industries are successful because they offer a quick, cheap, convenient meal that is high in; calories, fat, sugar and salt and low in fiber and calcium. Fast foods contain unhealthy fats that increase your risk of obesity, type 2 diabetes, high blood pressure and heart disease. Increased health risks are directly associated with fast foods, which is shown with the following individual study.

Morgan Spurlock is the man that ate a diet consisting of only McDonalds foods for 30 days straight Watch his documentary called Supersize me online. His experiment showed the following:

1. He gained 24.5 pounds.
2. His liver turned to fat
3. His cholesterol shot up 65 points.
4. He had an 11-15% body fat increase.
5. He nearly doubled his risk of coronary heart disease.
6. He became depressed and exhausted
7. His sex life was non-existent
8. He had bad mood swings
9. He had massive cravings and headaches.

"You do Deserve a Break Today," a break from illness. You stand no chance of healing if you continue to eat fast foods. These foods are a distant memory and at the bottom of the trashcan, along with lunch meats, hot dogs, sausage, bacon and scrapple, so scrap them!

Lunchmeats, Sausage, Bacon, Hotdogs, Scrapple

"Wonder" what's between the bread? Well you should. Before you make or grab a sandwich know that lunchmeats contain five dangerous additives and fillers. Cold cuts are a hot mess of chemicals, adding toxic trash to your body. *"Wish I was a whole lot leaner"* then you'll have to give up the wieners and the deli foods. The following are a list of some of the worst additives:

Corn syrup/Corn meal

This may upset your body's natural metabolism putting you at risk for obesity and also diabetes and heart disease. (Read more on simple sugars later in this chapter)

Listeria

Listeria does not discriminate between deli roast beef or pastrami. Unlike most bacteria, listeria germs can grow and spread in the refrigerator, including spreading to other foods. "*Listeria* has been linked to a variety of ready-to-eat foods, including deli meats, hot dogs, smoked foods, seafood and store-prepared deli-salads. A draft study released May 10, 2013 by the Food and Drug Administration (FDA) and the U.S. Department of Agriculture's Food Safety and Inspection Service (FSIS) evaluates the risk of listeria is associated with foods prepared in retail delis."

Sodium

Deli foods and salads contain iodized salt (sodium) which is used as a preservative. Sea salt is necessary for our bodily function, but often deli foods contain very large amounts of iodized salt. Sodium attracts water and a high-sodium diet draws water into the bloodstream, which increases the volume of blood and over time can increase your blood pressure. High blood pressure (also known as hypertension) forces the heart to work harder and can damage blood vessels and organs – increasing your risk of heart disease, kidney disease, and stroke.

Sodium Nitrate

This ingredient prevents the growth of botulism and alters the color of fish and meats. The combination of sodium nitrate and natural juices in meats, can be toxic for humans. It is dyed a pink color to avoid adding too much or confusing it for something else. Sodium nitrate is used as an ingredient in fertilizers, explosives, and glass and pottery enamels. Not good!

Added oils

It you look at the foods in the deli you will notice how they glisten. The meats and salads have a tempting shine because they are filled with a large amount of mayonnaise. The fats used in these pre-made salads can pack on some serious pounds quickly, not to mention add more toxins with the unhealthy selection of oil.

<u>Solution</u>: *Don't take a number at the deli!* Instead, cook organic meat at home and slice it up for lunch the next day.

Proteins
Meats

"Where's the Beef" hopefully not on your plate unless it is organic!!! Limit the beef, chicken and/or pork to a couple times a week. *"Meet your maker"* and purchase your meat at your local butcher shop where they do not use hormones or antibiotics. There are so many toxins in today's mass produced meat such as; antibiotics, growth hormones, mad cow, E. coli, salmonella, pink slime, Bovine Viral Diarrhea, and Meat Glue.

When I was a child, all the farms produced grass-fed beef and the cows were not slaughtered until they were at least 4-5 years old. Cattle have evolved for millions of years to eat grass, but now they are corn fed. Corn makes them sick so they are given antibiotics. You may be eating a sick, corn fed cow. Greed is the reason. It's faster, they are able to slaughter cows when they are less than 2 years old, making it more profitable. Sick, cheap, fast food...sound familiar? Start cleaning up your body, one organic hamburger or veggie burger at a time. Read more about the dangers of meat with antibiotics and hormones in Chapter 21.

"Old MacDonald had a Farm

And On This Farm He Had a Pig"
But Not Like This

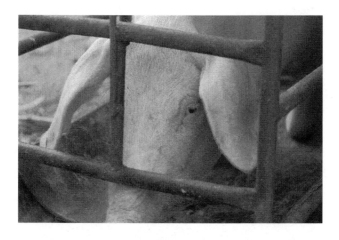

This is not how farm animals should be treated, but the truth is, this is how most un-organic pigs are raised. It makes me sick to my stomach to see how these precious animals are caged inside without sunlight. I am not condemning meat, but I ask everyone to buy their meat from an organic farm, where the animals are allowed to see the light of day, feed on grass and walk around on Gods great earth. What a cruel life; to stand or lie in a cage where they cannot even turn around. This also pertains to chickens, turkeys, calves, and cows.

"Milk Does Not Do a Body Good"

None of us want to hear this but, dairy is one of the most inflammatory foods in our diet. Hot, gooey, melted cheese is most delicious but is on the "naughty" list. Many of us are not aware of it, but most of the population cannot handle dairy. It causes inflammation resulting in digestive issues such as gas, bloating, constipation, and diarrhea. Some people are lactose intolerant; they have problems with the sugar found in milk. Others have problems with protein, the casein and whey. Casein has a molecular structure close to gluten. If that is not enough, know that if you are not drinking organic milk, you are consuming a mixed cocktail of chemicals, antibiotics and growth hormones. Read more in Chapter 21

Dairy Products to Avoid

- Butter and butter fat
- Cheese
- Cottage cheese
- Cream
- Sour cream and cream cheese
- All Milk, including buttermilk, powdered milk, and evaporated milk
- All Yogurt including Greek
- Ice cream
- Pudding

Fish Stories

Fish farming is the raising of fish commercially in tanks or enclosures in small spaces. There are also fish hatcheries when young fish are raised in a tank and then released into the wild to be recaptured at a later time. The most popular farm raised fish include, salmon, carp, tilapia and catfish. Farm raised fish and seafood equals a cesspool of toxic and dangerous chemicals you ingest through the food. Most supermarket fish is farm-raised, meaning that they use higher concentrates of antibiotics. Research has shown that farm raised fish also have a 20% lower protein content. Farm raised are given antibiotics to treat disease for overcrowded pool conditions. Sound familiar? It seems over-crowded habitats for farm animals produce the same results. There has been extensive commercialization and increased consumption of aquaculture seafood products worldwide.

The FDA is quoted as stating "Aqua-cultured seafood has become the fastest growing sector of the world food economy, accounting for approximately half of all seafood production worldwide. Approximately 80% of the seafood consumed in the U.S. is imported from approximately 62 countries. Over 40% of that seafood comes from aquaculture operations. As the aquaculture industry continues to grow and compete with wild-caught seafood products, concerns regarding the use of unapproved animal drugs and unsafe chemicals and the misuse of animal drugs in aquaculture operations have increased substantially." "China is the largest producer of aqua-cultured seafood in the world, accounting for 70% of the total production and 55% of the total value of aqua-cultured seafood exported around the world. The use of unapproved antibiotics or chemicals in aquaculture raises significant public health concerns."

"The FDA quoted on their website that studies show the seafood from China has a high percentage of contaminants and that in 2008 they were going to put a broader import control on all farm raised fish, shrimp, carp and eel from China." Don't wait, check the labels, and don't check out with farm raised fish, only wild caught.

No Peanuts or Peanut Butter

Two tablespoons of peanut butter packs around 190 calories, 135 of which come from both saturated and unsaturated fats. Peanuts are one of the most highly pesticide contaminated crops. Many people have severe allergy reactions to any products containing even trace amounts of peanuts. The worst reason is that peanuts mold easily and are often contaminated with aflatoxin. Aflatoxin is a mirotoxin that is produced from many different funguses.

Our government does sample testing of raw peanuts. The FDA has set maximum allowable aflatoxin in food commodities at 20 parts per billion (ppb); so minute amounts are allowable. They are tested when they are raw, and processing doesn't destroy the aflatoxin, so more can be growing in the peanut butter as it sits on the supermarket shelf. The following is a quote taken directly from the EPA site "Aflatoxin is the only mycotoxin regulated in America and is the most carcinogenic chemical known to science. If you have eaten 40 tablespoons of peanut butter, you have experienced a one in a million risk of dying from aflatoxin poisoning or an induced cancer. Many of us have eaten much more than this, so think about how we increase our risks by eating peanut butter.

"Beans, Beans the Poisonous Fruit"

Beans and other legumes are among the most nutritionally balanced foods. Beans are high in protein, complex carbohydrates, dietary fiber and many minerals and vitamins, while low in fat and cholesterol. However, beans contain a toxin called phytohemagglutinin (PHA) which is a member of the lectin family. Kidney beans in particular contain enough of this toxin to cause acute symptoms, even if only a few raw beans are eaten. PHA attacks and disables the epithelial cells lining the intestine and your body can get rid of them through severe vomiting and diarrhea. The safest bean is organic, no fat precooked beans or organic dry pinto beans soaked and cooked. Beans should never be eaten raw or sprouted and put on salads. Beans should always be soaked in water for several hours first, then discard the water, bring to a boil in fresh water and then cooked until done. By soaking beans and legumes for 2 hours and cooking them for ten minutes, most of the active lectins are eliminated.

FATS
Fried Foods

The next toxin to eliminate from our diets is something most of us really enjoy. They make us feel full and satisfied. Yes I'm talkin bout fried foods, *"Finger Lickin' Good"*. Frying foods can make anything taste good, even okra… yuck! Trans-fats are used in most fast food restaurants because they last longer than most conventional oils before they become rancid. Of course fast-food chains use different trans-fats in different locations. "For example, an analysis of samples of McDonald's French fries collected in 2004 and 2005 found that fries served in New York City contained twice as much trans-fat as in Hungary, and 28 times as much as in Denmark (where trans fats are restricted)."

Bad Fats (Eliminate)

Saturated fat	Trans fat
High-fat cuts of meat (beef, lamb, pork)	Packaged snack foods (crackers, microwave popcorn, chips)
Chicken with the skin	Stick margarine
Whole-fat dairy products (milk and cream)	Vegetable shortening
Butter	Fried foods (French fries, fried chicken, chicken nuggets, breaded fish)
Cheese	Candy bars
Ice cream	Commercially-baked pastries, cookies, doughnuts, muffins, cakes, pizza
Palm oil	
Lard	donuts

Sources of Trans-Fats

Many people think of margarine when they picture trans-fats, and it's true that some margarines are loaded with them. However, the primary source of trans-fats in the Western diet comes from commercially prepared baked goods and snack foods:

- **Baked goods** – cookies, crackers, cakes, muffins, pie crusts, pizza dough, and some breads like hamburger buns
- **Fried foods** – doughnuts, French fries, fried chicken, chicken nuggets, and hard taco shells
- **Snack foods** – potato, corn, and tortilla chips; candy; packaged or microwave popcorn
- **Solid fats** – stick margarine and semi-solid vegetable shortening
- **Pre-mixed products** – cake mix, pancake mix, and chocolate drink mix

When we eat the bad fats they increase our chances for chronic disease. These include saturated animal fats found in butter, lard, whole milk, ice cream, cream, cheese and high-fat meats like bacon. Plant-based fats that have been hydrogenated and contain trans-fat are found in margarines, shortenings, fried foods and commercial baked goods. These can also increase your risk for heart disease. "Burn fats not unhealthy oil."

Carbohydrates
Our Love Affair with Carbs

The fastest way to gain weight is to consume simple carbohydrates, which are not only very tasty but very addictive. When you eat carbs, your blood sugar rapidly rises. You get a temporary "high" when your blood sugar is high. Next, a blast of insulin from the pancreas causes a drop in blood sugar. At this point, feelings of weakness, fatigue, shakiness and even anxiety can set in. In order to feel good again, a person will indulge by eating another blast of carbs. This vicious cycle is exactly what happens to drug addicts/alcoholics, who must continue to have repeated "fixes" of their drug in order to feel good.

Besides, we all know that carbs are our comfort food. Carbs increase brain levels of tryptophan, which is the amino acid that converts to serotonin in the brain. Overeating Carbs, including breads, pastas, chips, and cookies, can temporarily help with depression, anxiety, and stress, giving us that instant lift we need. Most of us "self -medicate" due to cravings for these unhealthy carbs and sugars which leads to unhealthy weight gain.

A high-carb diet rich in simple carbohydrates, and lots of starches/breads, will cause you to gain weight which can contribute to insulin resistance and diabetes 2. When the blood glucose is too high, the pancreas becomes over-worked trying to produce enough insulin to compensate for the high blood glu-cose. Type 2 Diabetes occurs when there is too much fat on the blood cells and the pancreas doesn't produce enough insulin.

Other reasons for diabetes can be caused when the body is exhausted. My diet was almost perfect and I had diabetes. I also had adrenal fatigue so after a couple months of healing with supplements and detoxing, my diabetes disap-peared and has never returned.

See the correlation between overweight and obese individuals and diabetes in Chapter 10.

According to the American Diabetes Association, carbohydrates include the following three: *Complex carbohydrates (starches), simple carbohydrates (sugars) and fibers.*

Complex Carbs/starches (limit these)

Not all Carbs are created equal. The good part about complex carbs are that they digest slowly, prolong energy, are higher in fiber, and make us feel fuller longer. These carbs enter the blood stream slower and trigger only a moderate rise in insulin levels and help to have fewer carbs to be stored as fat.

The bad Complex carbohydrates include peas, corn, lima beans, white potatoes, and all grains including wheat, oats, pasta, corn, etc. However, the carbs listed below should be limited, Non GMO or eliminated for those who are having trouble losing weight and are ill with disease, disorders or food intolerances/allergies.

Complex Carbs - "a little dab'll do ya"

Bagel	Cereals	Jam
Baked beans	Cookies	Juice
Brown bread	Corn	Macaroni
Buck wheat	Cornmeal	Muesli
Cakes	Crackers	Multi-grain bread
Candy	High fiber cereals	Oat bran

- Oatmeal
- Pastas
- Peas
- Pita bread
- Potato
- Rice

- Soda
- Soy milk
- Soybeans
- Spaghetti
- Whole Barley

- Whole grain flours
- Whole meal bread
- Wild rice

White Foods/ Black list

The truth about white foods is that they are "the bad carbs;" white flour, white rice, white sugar and white salt. That means all pre-packaged junk food like cookies, cakes, candy, and pretzels are all on the bad list. So you need to kiss white foods goodbye if you want to lose weight and heal your illnesses. So what's all the hubbub about?

"White, Don't Bite It" White Flour

Bread, the *"slice of life"* just doesn't stack up in the health industry. What's the difference between white bread verses whole grain? Once the bread is stripped of the bran, the germ layers have been removed and the flour is bleached with chemicals such as potassium bromate or chlorine dioxide, you're left with a starch. Starch and Sugar are one in the same; they put you on a roller coaster high, only to crash and burn later. Then the cravings start and you want more and more. While white bread is so soft and light, and melts in your mouth, there are no nutrients in white bread products. The slogan should have been *"helps tear down your body 12 ways."* I know we could all just live and breathe bread and butter, not to mention its nurturing abilities.

So you don't *"knead the bread spread or the Levin rise,"* these go straight to your butt and gut, so leave the following alone:

- White Bread
- White Pasta
- White Wraps
- White Rice
- White Pizza Crust

- ❧ White Rolls
- ❧ White Muffins
- ❧ White Baked Goods
- ❧ White Bagels

Gluten Free Breads

Gluten free foods, breads, pastas and pastries, are a multibillion dollar industry and can be purchased in many restaurants and supermarkets. Gluten is the protein that is found in grains such as wheat, spelt, barley, oats and rye. Many people are gluten intolerant, have leaky gut syndrome, or celiac disease, where inflammation interferes with digestion. Gluten free does not necessarily mean healthy, meaning corn and rice can have damaging inflammatory effects on the body. Quinoa and amaranth also carry the label, but are high in saponins, which act as a defense mechanism for plants and can cause inflammation in the gut. Soy is a cheap grain and is genetically modified (GMO) and contains phytoestrogens which can wreak havoc on our bodies. The major problem with most gluten free products is that they contain refined sugar and unhealthy vegetable oils. *"Bake the Very Best"* Use only organic grain-free flour alternatives such as coconut, hazelnut and almond flours. These are my favorites and they contain protein and hardly any carbs. If you have a nut allergy then you will need to stay away from these.

"Rice a Phony" White Rice

Not such a treat! When rice is harvested, it first has the husk removed which leaves brown rice. Then the bran layer and germ are removed, along with the vitamins and minerals, making it white rice. Then a glucose layer is added to make it shine. It's not hair, just saying. If a product says enriched, it means quite the opposite. It is not "rich" it is actually a "poor" quality food; it has been robbed of its nutrients.

In the last ten years scientists have found high levels of arsenic in rice. Rice plants have the ability to absorb toxins from the soil more than any other grain. Arsenic has also been found in beer, when rice is used as an ingredient. It has also been found in rice beverages when used as a replacement for milk. Also, beware of brown rice syrup which is an additive in many products. Visit chapter 7 for more details on arsenic testing in rice.

Simple Carbohydrates/Sugar

In the 1800's people consumed about 18 pounds of sugar a year, in the 1900's 90 pounds of sugar, and in 2009 180 pounds of sugar. Sugar is in everything; soft drinks, fruit drinks, sauces, processed foods, canned foods, and you won't believe this one, most infant formula.....come on! Check it out yourself; most infant formulas contain sugar or corn syrup. No wonder kids are addicted to sugar so early in life.

There are naturally occurring sugars in fruits or milk (lactose). There are added sugars such as table sugar added to a cookie or heavy syrup which is added to canned fruit. There are so many different sugars such as table sugar, brown sugar, beet sugar, cane sugar, raw sugar, fruit sugar (fructose), turbinado, and high fructose corn syrup. Sounds like a song! Simple Sugars also include glucose (also known as dextrose), sucrose, fructose and galactose. The worst sugar is high fructose corn syrup, 55 percent fructose and 45 percent glucose. Simple carbs digest quickly, give a slow burst of energy, are low in fiber, make you hungry sooner and convert to fat cells.

High Fructose Corn Syrup (Stop Eating this or Gain Weight Fast)

Today, 55 percent of sweeteners used in food and beverage manufacturing are made from corn, and the number one source of calories in America's soda is, high fructose corn syrup. In the 1970's food and beverage manufacturers began switching their sweeteners from sucrose to corn syrup...why? Wait for it..... MONEY. They found out the high fructose corn syrup was much cheaper. It is also much sweeter than table sugar so they could use less. It doesn't stop there; studies have shown that it can lead more specifically to belly fat gain. Other health risks include elevated blood sugar, high blood pressure, elevated LDL, and decreased HDL, elevated triglycerides and non-alcohol fatty liver disease, which is alcohol without the buzz. It is time to totally eliminate high fructose corn syrup. Corn syrup tricks your body into gaining weight by fooling your metabolism. It turns off your body's appetite-control system, which results in an increased appetite to eat more. It does not appropriately stimulate insulin, which does not suppress the hunger hormone ghrelin. It also doesn't stimulate the satiety hormone leptin. So with this combination; you do not know when to stop eating and you do not feel full. And *"that's how the cookie crumbles."*

Sugar Alcohols are used in sugar-free candies. They include sorbitol, maltitol, xylitol, glycerol, erythritol and mannitol. They do not absorb completely into the small intestine so they have fewer calories than sugar but are known to cause diarrhea, flatulence and bloating.

Artificial Sweeteners are not sugars; they are chlorinated sweeteners, and very toxic chemicals. The following artificial sweeteners approved by the FDA include acesulfame, aspartame, saccharin, sucralose, and neotame. They are added to many baked goods and diet drinks to reduce the calories. However, just because they are approved does not mean they are healthy for you. Sucralose/Splenda in the yellow pack was marketed as being made from sugar, however, it is the same as aspartame (the blue pack) and saccharin (the pink pack); it is just another chemical.

Michael G. Tordoff, Department of Neurobiology, Physiology and Behavior, University of California at Davis, has published several studies showing that artificial sweeteners can:

1. increase hunger, short-term food intake, and cravings
2. affect blood sugar levels, which can be especially dangerous to people with diabetes or epilepsy
3. cause fluid retention
4. increase cellulite
5. contribute to weight gain

In one study, he found that aspartame in chewing gum increased hunger due to oral stimulation by the added chemicals. His study also showed a gender-related sweetness response, which explains why certain people feel "ravenous" after consuming aspartame-containing products, while others do not.

White Sugar

Simple carbs/white sugars are empty calories, no nutritional value at all and are very dangerous carbs. When broken down and digested quickly, they leave you feeling tired, hungry, and craving more sugar shortly after you've eaten. Recent research has shown that certain simple carbohydrate foods can cause extreme surges in blood sugar levels, which also increases insulin release. This can elevate appetite and the risk of excess fat storage. Simply stay away from Simple Carbs! There are health risks that include the risk of obesity, diabetes, cardiovascular disease, gout in men and metabolic syndrome.

"Things Do Not go Better with Coke"

"Coke Adds Life" Are you kidding me. How far from the truth is this? Here is where some will draw the line, thinking there is no way they can give up their soda's and so called energy drinks. Soda Pop, Energy Drinks, Sports drinks and Fruit Juice are nothing more than a heaping cup of chemicals. I am sorry to say but you *"can't have it your way"* here. They must go. A substitute is Vitamin Max B from Premier Research Lab. It will instantly give you more energy without the sugar, corn syrup and caffeine. In the United States:

63 million people consume diet soda
158 million people consume sugar drinks

Wow! We can all agree that soda/drinks are high in calories and sugar and low in nutrients. Soda contributes to obesity, tooth decay, weakens bones and starts caffeine dependence. Studies show that people have an unhealthy diet to go along with this. We already know that sugar makes us fat, but did you know sugar drinks have a pH of only 2.9 which is highly acidic. This has been called the melting pot by many dentists, as when you bathe your teeth in a citric acid and the sugar combo it breaks down the tissue, bone and teeth. I knew this at a very early age as I chewed about two packs of gum a day, back when gum came in a five pack. I had 16 cavities at one time, and had ten of those removed in the last two years.

Caffeine is a stimulant, that's right, like cocaine and tobacco, and it is considered a drug, which is why we become dependent on it. Have you ever tried to give up your cup of java? If so you will notice detox/withdrawal symptoms; headaches, irritability, and a rise in blood pressure. Soda with sugar contains about 35 to 38 milligrams of caffeine per 12 ounce can, but did you know that diet soda packs in about 42 milligrams of caffeine. Diet soda is even a worse choice since the artificial sugar is a chemical and it contains more caffeine to boot.

Lose Energy with Energy Drinks

Most energy drinks claim to be a magic potion of vitamins and minerals to boost energy. Many have guarana, taurine, ginseng, and synthetic B vitamins made from coal tar. The manufacturers are not required to list whether the herbs have been sprayed with pesticides, or if they are synthetically made. Most sports and energy drinks contain the following; Sugar, Dextrose, Citric Acid, MSG, Natural Flavor, Salt, Sodium Citrate, Monopotassium, Phosphate, Gum Arabic, Sucrose, Acetate Isobutyrate, Glycerol, Ester of Rosin, and Yellow 6.

Three ounces of sugar in any form like: fruit juice, soda or sport drinks, suppress the activity of white blood cells for up to 5 hours. It's estimated that Americans drink 22% of their total calories, from beverages sweetened with sugar, high-fructose corn syrup and artificial sweeteners.

"Good to the Last Drop" Coffee

Many people will agree with that; they love their coffee. Coffee contains caffeine, which artificially speeds up your body. You should be able to wake up and have energy on your own. Do you find that you need more and more coffee to make it through your day? Try to limit your coffee to a cup in the morning and make sure it is organic. "Don't be fooled that it is "mountain grown." Coffee is the heaviest chemically treated food in the world. Heavy synthetic nitrogen fertilizers are used when growing coffee. Human health concerns surrounding contamination include certain cancers, birth defects, blue baby syndrome, hypertension and developmental problems in children. Coffee is grown slowly in the rain forest, which like everything else in the world is too slow. So to speed up the process, 70 percent of the coffee bean is now grown in the sun as a resistant hybrid. Moldiness in green coffee may occur during curing, drying, and storage periods. Water damage of bagged coffee may also promote the growth of molds on the beans. The major pest attacking coffee beans is the coffee berry borer beetle. So make the *"best part of waking up is"* Premiers Max B in your cup.

White Salt

Iodized salt just may be the *"salt of the earth,"* but through better judgment, can be replaced with Pink Sea Salt from the "salt of the sea." Almost every client I see will tell me they do not use salt because they think salt is unhealthy for them. They are right about table/white iodized salt because it is produced by taking natural tan colored salt (or crude oil flake leftovers) and heating it up to 1200° Fahrenheit turning it into a white chemical.

What's so dangerous is that Iodized salt is in almost every prepackaged food that we eat. Salt is used as a preservative, and on a food item, it can kill living bacteria. Very few companies are using sea salt because of the expense and yes…Greed! Medical doctors will also insist that you do not use iodized salt because it can raise blood pressure very quickly since the blood is attempting to move toxins rapidly away from the heart. It also can be very damaging to the digestive system, cause dehydration, and retention of water, which can lead to increased problems for diabetes, gout and obesity.

The level of white salt in prepackaged foods is so high that over time it can cause destruction to major organs. Salt is also highly addictive, meaning the more you use, the more you want. This also leads us to a midnight snack, craving a salty snack such as potato chips and pretzels.

3

"IT'S THE REAL THING" LIVE FOOD

The Good Carbs

This list contains a group of foods that should be eaten daily. As you can see there are mostly fruits and vegetables which are antioxidants and protect the body since they contain many vitamins and minerals. Antioxidants protect cells against free radical damage which cause disease. Antioxidants that protect against these diseases include beta-carotene, lutein, lycopene, selenium, vitamin A, vitamin C and vitamin E.

- Avocado
- Bananas
- Beans
- Broccoli
- Brown Rice
- Brussels Sprouts
- Cabbage
- Carrots
- Cassava
- Cauliflower
- Celery
- Chickpeas
- Cucumbers
- Dill Pickles
- Dried Apricots
- Eggplant
- Garbanzo Beans
- Grapefruit
- Kidney Beans
- Lentils
- Lettuce
- Navy Beans
- Okra
- Onions
- Oranges
- Pinto Beans

- Plums
- Prunes
- Radishes
- Spinach
- Split peas
- Sprouts
- Strawberry
- Sweet Potato
- Tomatoes
- Turnip Greens
- Watercress
- Yam
- Zucchini

Fats
Good Fats

Monounsaturated fat
- Olive oil
- Canola oil
- Sunflower oil
- Sesame oil
- Avocados
- Olives
- Nuts (almonds, macadamia nuts, hazelnuts, pecans, cashews)

Polyunsaturated fat
- Non GMO Soybean oil
- Safflower oil
- Walnuts
- Sunflower, sesame, and pumpkin seeds
- Flaxseed
- Fatty fish (salmon, tuna, mackerel, herring, trout, sardines)
- Non GMO Soymilk, Tofu

"Good Fats" are monounsaturated and polyunsaturated fats.

- May help reduce risk factors of heart disease and stroke
- May help reduce risk of diabetes
- Could promote healthy nerve activity
- Are shown to improve vitamin absorption
- Are required to maintain healthy immune system
- Promote cell development, they help lower levels of bad cholesterol, increase your good cholesterol
- Help to prevent inflammation.

These fats are liquid at room temperature. Eating healthy fats, in moderation, during weight loss fulfills your dietary fat needs without increasing your chronic disease risks. Examples of heart-healthy fats include plant-based oils, such as **olive, walnut, and flaxseed oils, nuts, seeds, nut butters, avocados and olives. Nuts and seeds** are rich in heart-healthy fats as well as fiber and protein, which increase satiety more than carbs or fat, so they are an ideal choice when you're trying to shed pounds. Do not choose the unhealthy oils such as peanut, corn, canola and soybean oil. There are better choices. If you must use corn oil or soybean, make sure it is Non GMO.

Omega-3 fatty acids

Omega-3 fatty acids help cognitive function, memory, problem-solving abilities, help you battle fatigue, sharpen your memory, and balance your mood. Omega-3 fats are a type of essential fatty acid, meaning they are essential to health, but your body can't make them. You can only get omega-3 fats from food.

- DHA – Docosahexaenoic acid (DHA) have the most research to back up their health benefits. Found in abundance in cold-water fatty fish or purchase DHA from Premier Research.
- ALA – Alpha-linolenic acid (ALA) comes from plants. Studies suggest that it's a less potent form of omega-3 than EFA and DHA. The best sources include flaxseed, walnuts, and canola oil.

The best sources are fatty fish such as salmon (especially wild-caught king and sockeye), herring, mackerel, anchovies, or sardines. Canned albacore tuna and lake trout can also be good sources, depending on how the fish were raised and processed. If you're a vegetarian or you don't like fish, you can still get your omega-3 fix by eating algae (which is high in DHA) or taking an algae supplement.

"Think Pink" Pink Salt

Use pink salt every day. Our organs, adrenals, cells, even tissues in our bodies actually need healthy salt to keep us hydrated, help with digestion and thyroid, and balance our sodium potassium levels, bone density, circulation and stabilization of blood sugar. So salt is good for us....repeat this ten times!

So now that we have determined that we do need salt, let's take a look at the healthy salt. The color of the salt should be pink so that you can see that it actually still has the powerful minerals still included. Use Himalayan pink salt from the mountains or Pink Salt from the ocean. I prefer the pink salt from Premier Research Labs. It is hand dried naturally in the sun. Depending on your lifestyle, you need to consume at least half a teaspoon a day. This sounds like a lot, but I promise you your body will thank you.

Healthier Sugars

Raw Honey is natural in its raw form. It is about 53 percent fructose. Honey is probably one of the healthiest of the sugars as it contains many antioxidants. Make sure it is raw and organic.

Stevia comes from the stevia plant in South America. It is a natural sweetener and considered to be a safe sugar alternative. Some people do not like it because they think it is too sweet and it has an after taste.

Coconut Sugar is a great choice and contains trace amounts of vitamin C, B, potassium, phosphorous, magnesium, calcium, zinc, iron and copper. Coconut sugar also provides small amounts of phytonutrients, and antioxidants. You'll also find the B vitamin inositol, often used as a mood booster in coconut sugar. The glycemic index measures the carbohydrates in your blood. Coconut sugar ranks 35 on this index compared to sugar at 60.

Agave Syrup is a sweetener that comes from the blue agave plant. The only ingredient is agave, but it can be highly processed like corn syrup. It is very sweet and has 60 calories per tablespoon compared to 40 for table sugar. Make sure you purchase raw organic Agave and just use a small amount.

Raw Fruits/fructose are the healthiest choice. On the next page you will find a chart of fruits that list the serving size, total fructose, carbs, sugars, vitamins and fiber. Even though fresh fruit contains fructose it is still healthy than eating sugar or drinking fruit juice. The fresh fruit contains fiber and is loaded with antioxidants. So enjoy some fruit each day.

Experiment with raw sweeteners. These are generally made from pureed sweet fruits, such as dates. If these foods satisfy your sweet tooth, they are much more nutritionally dense and less caloric than traditional sweeteners, and will definitely help you lose weight.

Fiber

Fiber is the indigestible part of plant foods, including vegetables, whole grains, fruits, nuts and legumes. When you consume these fibers, most of it passes through the intestines like Roto Rooter, cleaning out your digestive track. Fiber helps to make you feel full and satisfied after eating. Additional health benefits of a diet high in fiber include a reduction in cholesterol levels.

"Sometimes You Feel Like a Nut"

Nuts are a great way to add protein and good fat into a nutritious snack. The best way to eat nuts is to make sure they are organic and raw. When anything is cooked it loses some of the nutrients. You do not want to eat nuts that are candy-coated, fried in oil or covered in iodized salt. You will need to avoid peanuts because of the containments and mold factor.

The best and healthiest way to prepare your nuts is to soak the nuts in water for 2 hours in a glass bowl. The only nut that does not need to be soaked is cashews. After soaking nuts you will notice that much of the residue and tannins are released into the water leaving a milder, softer more buttery nut flavor. Also, nuts and seeds will release toxic enzyme inhibitors and reduce phytic acid. Lastly, place them in a colander and rinse, put them in a dehydrator and add some pink salt until nuts are dry. By soaking nuts and seeds, you release these toxic enzyme inhibitors and increase the life and vitality contained within them!

The Benefits of Soaking Nuts and Seeds

- Enzyme inhibitors get neutralized.
- The amount of vitamins your body can absorb increases.
- Phytic acid, which inhibits the absorption of vital minerals, is reduced.

Fruits

Nutrition Facts

Raw, edible weight portion. Percent Daily Values (%DV) are based on a 2,000 calorie diet.

Fruits — Serving Size (gram weight/ounce weight)	Calories	Calories from Fat	Total Fat (g)	Total Fat %DV	Sodium (mg)	Sodium %DV	Potassium (mg)	Potassium %DV	Total Carbohydrate (g)	Total Carb %DV	Dietary Fiber (g)	Dietary Fiber %DV	Sugars (g)	Protein (g)	Vitamin A %DV	Vitamin C %DV	Calcium %DV	Iron %DV
Apple — 1 large (242 g/8 oz)	130	0	0	0	0	0	260	7	34	11	5	20	25g	1g	2%	8%	2%	2%
Avocado — California, 1/5 medium (30 g/1.1 oz)	50	35	4.5	7	0	0	140	4	3	1	1	4	0g	1g	0%	4%	0%	2%
Banana — 1 medium (126 g/4.5 oz)	110	0	0	0	0	0	450	13	30	10	3	12	19g	1g	2%	15%	0%	2%
Cantaloupe — 1/4 medium (134 g/4.8 oz)	50	0	0	0	20	1	240	7	12	4	1	4	11g	1g	120%	80%	2%	2%
Grapefruit — 1/2 medium (154 g/5.5 oz)	60	0	0	0	0	0	160	5	15	5	2	8	11g	1g	35%	100%	4%	0%
Grapes — 3/4 cup (126 g/4.5 oz)	90	0	0	0	15	1	240	7	23	8	1	4	20g	0g	0%	2%	2%	0%
Honeydew Melon — 1/10 medium melon (134 g/4.8 oz)	50	0	0	0	30	1	210	6	12	4	1	4	11g	1g	2%	45%	2%	2%
Kiwifruit — 2 medium (148 g/5.3 oz)	90	10	1	2	0	0	450	13	20	7	4	16	13g	1g	2%	240%	4%	2%
Lemon — 1 medium (58 g/2.1 oz)	15	0	0	0	0	0	75	2	5	2	2	8	2g	0g	0%	40%	2%	0%
Lime — 1 medium (67 g/2.4 oz)	20	0	0	0	0	0	75	2	7	2	2	8	0g	0g	0%	35%	0%	0%
Nectarine — 1 medium (140 g/5.0 oz)	60	5	0.5	1	0	0	250	7	15	5	2	8	11g	1g	8%	15%	0%	2%
Orange — 1 medium (154 g/5.5 oz)	80	0	0	0	0	0	250	7	19	6	3	12	14g	1g	2%	130%	6%	0%
Peach — 1 medium (147 g/5.3 oz)	60	0	0.5	1	0	0	230	7	15	5	2	8	13g	1g	6%	15%	0%	2%
Pear — 1 medium (166 g/5.9 oz)	100	0	0	0	0	0	190	5	26	9	6	24	16g	1g	0%	10%	2%	0%
Pineapple — 2 slices, 1" diameter, 3/4" thick (112 g/4 oz)	50	0	0	0	10	0	120	3	13	4	1	4	10g	1g	2%	50%	2%	2%
Plums — 2 medium (151 g/5.4 oz)	70	0	0	0	0	0	230	7	19	6	2	8	16g	1g	8%	10%	0%	2%
Strawberries — 8 medium (147 g/5.3 oz)	50	0	0	0	0	0	170	5	11	4	2	8	8g	1g	0%	160%	2%	2%
Sweet Cherries — 21 cherries; 1 cup (140 g/5.0 oz)	100	0	0	0	0	0	350	10	26	9	1	4	16g	1g	2%	15%	2%	2%
Tangerine — 1 medium (109 g/3.9 oz)	50	0	0	0	0	0	160	5	13	4	2	8	9g	1g	6%	45%	4%	0%
Watermelon — 1/18 medium melon; 2 cups diced pieces (280 g/10.0 oz)	80	0	0	0	0	0	270	8	21	7	1	4	20g	1g	30%	25%	2%	4%

Most fruits provide negligible amounts of saturated fat, *trans* fat, and cholesterol; avocados provide 0.5 g of saturated fat per ounce.

U.S. Food and Drug Administration
(January 1, 2008)

NUTS &SEEDS

	PROTEIN	CARB	FIBER	Sat. Fat	Mono Fat	ω-3 Fat	ω-6 Fat	Calories
ALMOND	6.0	6.1	3.5	1.1	8.8	0.2	3.4	163
BRAZIL	4.1	3.5	2.1	4.3	7.0	0.05	5.8	186
CASHEW	5.2	8.6	0.9	2.2	6.7	0.2	2.2	157
PEANUT	7.0	4.5	2.4	1.9	6.8	0	4.4	159
HAZELNUT	4.2	4.7	2.7	1.3	12.9	0.24	2.2	178
MACADEMIA	2.2	3.9	2.4	3.4	16.7	0.06	0.36	204
PECAN	2.6	3.9	2.7	1.8	11.6	0.28	5.8	196
PISTACHIO	5.8	7.8	2.9	1.6	6.8	0.71	3.7	159
WALNUT	4.3	3.9	1.9	1.7	2.5	2.5	10.7	185
PINE	3.8	3.7	1.0	1.4	5.3	0.31	9.4	188
PUMPKIN	9.3	5.0	1.1	2.4	4.0	0.51	5.8	151
FLAX	1.8	8.1	7.6	1.0	2.1	6.3	1.7	150
CHIA	4.4	12.3	10.6	0.9	0.6	4.9	1.6	137
SESAME	5.0	6.6	3.3	1.9	5.3	0.11	6.0	160
SUNFLOWER	5.5	5.6	2.4	1.2	5.2	0.21	6.5	164

4

"THINGS GO BETTER WITH" GOOD DIGESTION

Healthy Digestion is one of the best ways to heal ourselves and to lose weight. This will include drinking water, adding sea salt, taking good quality oils, eating foods high in fiber and using probiotics.

"As your Stomach Turns" What not to eat

Do you suffer from stomach pain, ulcers, reflux, constipation, gas, Crohn's disease, Inflammatory Bowel Syndrome (IBS), Colitis, Celiac Disease, etc? Many people suffer daily with these uncomfortable and embarrassing symptoms. Many are on the wrong diet. You will need to eliminate the junk and add in the fiber. It will take time if you have any of the above issues, because it will start to clean out the digestive system which can cause stomach pain, gas or diarrhea. Many people will stop because of this, when they really need to just stick with it. Remember to add these foods slowly to avoid uncomfortable symptoms. This is where the cure lies.

For healthy digestion, you will need to eliminate all junk food, fast food, most grains, sugar, sodas and fruit drinks, white flour products, frozen foods, processed foods, boxed foods, ice cream, cakes and cookies, even dairy including yogurt. Many people are allergic to the above listed foods, because, here it comes again, too many toxins. Once you are able to turn digestion on and rid your body of toxins, you will be able to bring some of the foods back. If you decide to stay on dairy, make sure it is organic. Purchase an organic Greek yogurt that has no sugar or fruit on the bottom, adding only your own organic fruit. For now, I would rather you give dairy up during your initial detox period.

"Nothing But Pure Refreshment" Drink More Water

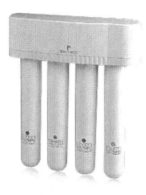

Women and Men need to drink an adequate amount of water. It is best to drink your own water from home. You may want to obtain a municipal water report, testing for lead, mercury, nitrates, E-coli and bacteria. This report is yours by law and most states offer the test at a very inexpensive price. Most people are going to need to start using a filtration system. The most inexpensive would be to use one of the drip water filter systems that filter into a pitcher. The next step up would be to install a filter system under your kitchen sink to use for drinking water. You will also need to add a filtered shower nozzle. Many people do not realize that when you jump into a warm shower you are opening up your pores and allowing all of those chemicals to enter and contaminate your body. For those fortunate families, it is best to install a whole house system. Below is a very affordable system from Premier Research Labs. Keep you and your family safe with a reverse osmosis filtration system.

Trust the Water in Your Home

Water Purifiers

Purchase a reverse osmosis filtration system for clean and healthy drinking water. Our bodies are made up of 55-60% water, and drinking healthy, purified water is crucial to living a happy and energetic life. This system is designed to fit underneath your sink, so it is out of sight but never out of mind.

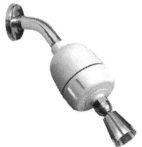

Shower Filters

Experience an energy-enhanced shower with a filter that converts chlorine into a harmless soluble chloride for better lathering with healthier water. Without a filter a hot shower turns the chlorine into a gaseous vapor that contaminates our skin, as well as our respiratory system, kidneys, and various other organs in our bodies.

The good news is that everywhere you go you see people walking around drinking water. However, the majority are carrying water in toxic water bottles. The problem with bottled water is twofold; the quality of the water in the bottle and the plastic bottle itself. Unless a bottle is marked BPA free, it contains the toxins BPA. BPA stands for bisphenol A. BPA is an industrial chemical that has been used to make certain plastics and resins since the 1960s. BPA is found in polycarbonate plastics and epoxy resins. Polycarbonate plastics are often used in containers that store food and beverages, such as water bottles and metal cans. Some research has shown that BPA can seep into food or beverages from containers that are made with BPA. There are some health concerns with BPA having negative effects on the brain, behavior and prostate gland of fetuses, infants and children.

The Food and Drug Administration (FDA) has stated that BPA is safe at the very low levels that occur in some foods. However, at the same time gives the following suggestions from their website:

Here is information for consumers who want to limit their exposure to BPA:

- Plastic containers have recycle codes on the bottom. Some, but not all, plastics that are marked with recycle codes 3 or 7 may be made with BPA.
- Do not put very hot or boiling liquid that you intend to consume in plastic containers made with BPA. BPA levels rise in food when containers/products made with the chemical are heated and come in contact with the food.
- Discard all bottles with scratches, as these may harbor bacteria and, if BPA-containing, lead to greater release of BPA.

They openly admit not to put hot liquids into plastic made with BPA. Another thing to consider is to never buy your bottled water where it is sitting out in the hot sun. Have you ever drive up to a gas station and see cases of water just sitting out in the sun heating up the chemicals inside?

Buy Glass! Glass is your best option or purchase BPA free plastic containers. They are clearly marked on the bottles.

How much water do you need? Every system in your body needs water. Water is one way to flush the toxins out of the organs. It also carries nutrients to your cells. We lose water through urine, bowel movements and perspiration. Men need about 12 cups (96 ounces) a day where women need about 8 cups, (64 ounces) a day. If you are drinking herbal hot or cold tea beverages with no additives such as sugar, this can be counted as part of your water consumption.

"When It Rains, It Pours" Salt

The next step is to add pink sea salt. Most of you have been told that salt is not good for you. You may have been told that it causes fluid retention. Iodized salt or table salt is not good for the human body because it is heated above 1,200 degrees, changing its chemical structure which means you are ingesting a chemical toxin. This cheap salt also can contain anti-caking agents, which makes it easier to pour and aluminum. So toss the iodized salt or save it to put down on your walk ways when it snows. Iodized salt is acid forming to the body, whereas sea salt produces an alkalizing effect. Iodine is important for hormone health. Since there is only a small amount of iodine in sea salts, alternatives include eating seaweed, cod, shrimp and eggs. Premier Pink Salt, from PRL, is organic raw sea salt from prehistoric, unpolluted sea beds. This natural, sun-dried sea salt contains unheated trace minerals in addition to unheated sodium chloride. These minerals, undamaged by heat, retain their high energy, are ideal for helping to maintain fluid balance in the body. Its rich trace mineral content gives it a slightly pink color. It is composed of tiny mineral rich crystals formed millions of years before pollution contaminated our present oceans.

"The Sign of Good Taste" Oils

Fat is essential for normal growth and development of our bodies. It is not something we want to eliminate from our diet. Good fat provides energy, maintains cell membranes, protects our organs and helps the body to absorb nutrients. Women's bodies were created to hold more body fat than men because of the child bearing years. When women do not ingest good oils and water, this can cause sagging breasts, stretch marks, dry and hard bowel movements and dry skin.

All fats are not created equal. It takes fat to burn fat. So many of us think that limiting fat intake will help us to lose weight...Wrong! It is actually the opposite; we need GOOD fats (refer to chapter 3 for the list) to lose weight. I would suggest an intake of Premiers Research Labs Essential Fatty Acid (EFA) oil at least 1 teaspoon by mouth or 4 caps a day along with 1 tablespoon of Premiers Coconut oil and 5 DHA caps daily. Avocados are a fabulous healthy fat to add to our diet. Be careful with most EFA oil purchases because many of them are made from fish oils. Remember, most of the fish are farm raised and you are defeating your purpose by just adding more toxins to your body.

So let's just keep it easy. Eat a small amount of good carbs and the body will burn those carbs, eat a little bit of good fat and the body will burn that fat. Eat large amounts of bad carbs with bad fat, like a pizza, and you will gain weight. My motto: Balance and moderation. I believe the body needs a balance of carbs, proteins, and fat for the body to function. Example: eating pizza (carb bread, cheese protein and fat) verses eating a salad with an avocado and beans (carb salad, avocado fat, and protein beans). Sure who does not want to devour a pizza...it feels so good, but then an hour later we start to suffer with bloating and pain. *"Only you can prevent weight gain."* Put fire in your body with the good foods and let it burn the fat. You decide! Do you want to feel good, look good and be healthy or eat whatever you want and suffer the consequences. *"Don't let your stomach become a waste basket."*

"Add the Pickles, Add the Lettuce" Fiber

What has no calories and it's not water? And the answer is...fiber. Fiber does not contain any calories because the digestive enzymes in your body do not digest fiber. Another great reason to consume fiber is that it helps you to feel full due to the absorption of water and because it takes longer to chew most fiber foods, vegetables and fruits. Dietary fiber, known as roughage, includes all parts of plant foods that your body can't digest or absorb. Dietary fiber is found mainly in four groups: fruits, vegetables, whole grains and nuts, seeds & legumes (beans). Fiber passes relatively intact through your stomach, small intestine, colon and then out of your body. There are two types of fiber; soluble (dissolves in water) and insoluble (does not dissolve in water). Both types of fiber are equally important for health, digestion, and preventing conditions such as diabetes, heart disease, obesity, diverticulitis, and constipation. Fiber will increase the size, weight and bulk of your stool making it easier to have a bowel movement. It can also firm up a loose watery stool too.

Soluble Fiber

Soluble fiber forms a gel in the digestive tract, and slows digestion and prevents the body from absorbing too much starch and sugar. Soluble fiber delays the emptying of your stomach and makes you feel full, which helps control weight. It can help lower blood cholesterol and glucose levels.

Sources of natural soluble fiber: Make you feel full, slow digestion

- oatmeal
- lentils
- apples
- barley
- oranges
- pears

- oat bran
- strawberry
- nuts
- flaxseeds
- beans
- dried peas

- blueberry
- psyllium
- cucumbers
- celery/ carrots

Insoluble fiber

This type of gut-healthy fiber promotes the movement of material through your digestive system, like a laxative effect, and increases stool bulk, so it can be of benefit to those who struggle with constipation or irregular stools. Insoluble fiber does not dissolve in water so food passes through the digestive tract and speeds up the passage of food and waste products.

Sources of Natural Insoluble Fiber

- Seeds
- Nuts
- Barley
- Couscous
- Brown rice

- Bulgur
- Zucchini
- Celery
- Broccoli
- Cabbage

- Cauliflower
- Onions
- Tomatoes
- Carrots
- Cucumbers
- Green beans
- Dark leafy vegetables
- Fruit
- Root vegetable
- Skins (potatoes)
- Whole grains
- Wheat bran

Don't worry about counting fiber or deciding which group of fiber you need. Focus on eating a healthy diet, rich in four of the fiber groups: fruits, vegetables, legumes, nuts, & seeds. This will provide a variety of soluble and insoluble fibers and all of the health benefits. Although whole wheat breads and grains have fiber, they are to be avoided as much as possible. If you have irritable bowel syndrome, celiac disease, colitis, Crohn's or are Gluten Intolerant avoid all grains. *"I'd walk a mile for a piece of bread."* I don't know about you, but if I eat bread or pasta, I have a hard time with portion control and wanting more and more. Limit or eliminate bread and pasta. If you do need to use bread, make sure it is whole grain wheat bread or whole grain pasta. A better substitute would be to use some brown rice instead.

Also, as you change your diet and incorporate more fiber, most people will experience more intestinal gas. Make sure to add Premiers HCL into your diet after you eat and drink more water to help the digestive process. Your body will adapt, just know that your body is detoxing and clearing out your colon. Relief is on its way and you will be able to eat fibrous food eventually without the gas.

What is colon hydrotherapy?

Colon hydrotherapy is a gentle, natural method of washing acquired wastes from the entire colon. When completed, the body no longer has to deal with waste that has been accumulated during a lifetime, which prevents the body from healing itself and fighting disease. Virtually everyone has these built-up wastes in their colon, especially from eating processed and fast foods. Colon hydrotherapy helps a person lose toxic waste which then increases the body's metabolic rate. People have been known to lose up to 10 pounds after just one appointment. Research in America and Europe has shown that people can carry from 10 to 50 pounds of accumulated toxic material, with the majority stored in the colon.

The purpose of colon hydrotherapy is to clean and flush away-unwanted toxins, however; it will not fully correct its underlying causes. Colon hydrotherapy only serves as the first step to healing. Cleansing paired with nutritional support may help the colon return to its normal bowel functions. Restoring power to the colon requires the body's digestive wastes to be eliminated.

Some Ailments that May be Relieved by Colon Hydrotherapy:

❧ Allergies	❧ Indigestion
❧ Bursitis	❧ Headaches
❧ Constipation	❧ Lack of Energy
❧ Colitis	❧ Bloating
❧ Digestive Issues	❧ Parasites
❧ Fatigue	❧ Skin Disorders
❧ Food Sensitivities	❧ Swelling in legs

The best place to start and solve most irregular bowel functions requires a combination of some of these products from Premier Research Labs.

HCL - 100% natural-source betaine hydrochloride, created to assist the body's natural stomach acids in the digestion and absorption of nutrients, especially protein, vitamin B12, calcium, iron and other minerals. As we age, we typically produce less hydrochloric acid (HCL) which reduces our ability to efficiently absorb nutrients from food. Reduced HCL production affects the amount of protein and calcium we can absorb and can interfere with bone metabolism.

Digest Premier - This formula is highly effective for digestive support as well as cleansing. Help to digest cooked food.

Digestase - This extraordinary plant-based enzyme formula supports the digestion of carbohydrates and protein and is helpful for vegetarians and those gluten-intolerant.

Probiotics - The broad-spectrum, premier probiotic formula (with "good bacteria") promotes healthy intestinal ecology with 12 different viable strains of beneficial flora to support health-promoting intestinal bacteria. Our unique fermentation process uses 95 different natural herbs and barks, cultured for 3 years to produce healthy, mature flora and highly bioavailable nutrients.

Galactan™ delivers great-tasting, fiber-rich nutrition with arabinogalactan from the Larch tree that supports optimal immune system integrity as well as healthy bowel regularity and gastrointestinal health. It also supports beneficial gastrointestinal microflora. Great addition to smoothies or other drinks.

When our intestinal tract is irritated, toxic fats are not processed correctly and they begin to enter the large intestines. The healthy bile in our large intestines absorbs the fat soluble toxins that it finds and boosts our immune system. Most of us are aware that 70 percent of our immune system is in our gut/colon. The large intestines can absorb heavy metals, parasites, pesticides, bad bacteria and numerous other cancer and disease causing chemicals. Toxins are not eliminated with the stool, instead these toxins remain in the colon and some are reabsorbed back to the liver. The more toxic the liver, the more toxic the intestines, makes it harder to break down the everyday toxins such as meat, food additives, etc. The liver is unable to handle the toxic fat cells, and the bile is too sluggish to buffer the stomach acid that enters the small intestines. This is when many people are unable to handle most foods, because they are so toxic.

"Plop plop, Fizz fizz, Oh What a Relief it is" Probiotics

Probiotics are organisms containing live bacteria or yeast that supplements normal gastrointestinal flora. The healthy flora becomes depleted by infections, antibiotic use and ingesting toxic foods over time. There are over 500 different types of bacteria which help keep our intestines healthy and boost our immune system. Probiotics are an essential part of regaining good intestinal flora, improving the lining of the intestines. Many people use fermented dairy products, such as yogurt and kefir, because they contain live bacteria. However, most of the dairy products still contain antibiotics and hormones and most people are unable to tolerate dairy. So I am recommending a probiotic verses dairy products. I suggest Premier Research Labs Probiotic.

Correlation Between Meat Consumption and Colon Cancer Rates in Different Countries

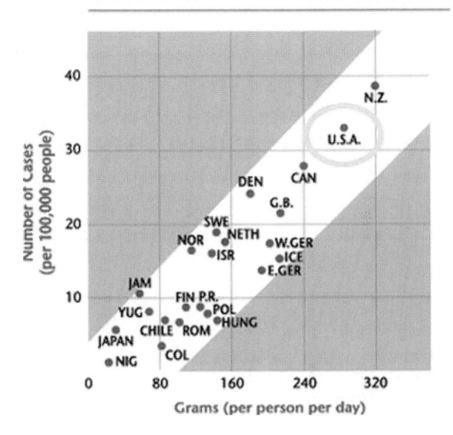

This is an interesting graph showing the more meat consumed the higher rate of colon cancer. As you can see, New Zealand consumed the most meat and had the highest number of colon cancer with the United States being the second highest. This graph is courtesy of the China Study, which is a great reference book for recommended reading, filled with information on cancers.

Damage to your digestive tract heads the list of priorities for stubborn weight issues and causes an increase in cravings for sugar, carbohydrates and/or high calorie foods. A digestive problem/inflammation/toxicity interferes with the body's metabolism and will slow your ability to lose weight. Many people have increased belly fat just because they are carrying a lot of toxic impacted food in their colons.

Antibiotic use can greatly interfere with our digestive system, usually giving women a yeast infection or Candida Albicans. Women that use a lot of antibiotics can be at risk for major digestive problems such as leaky gut, IBS, etc. The problem with antibiotics is that they come into the body and attack bacteria everywhere, not just a specific infection. The antibiotics don't discriminate between which bacteria, and wreak havoc on the good bacteria in your intestinal track. A depressed immune system can subsequently cause food cravings; and many do not even know why they are having these cravings. Antibiotics and high sugar consumption, carbs, junk food and alcohol also lead to an imbalanced overgrowth of Candida albicans. If you have Candida, you will need to follow the candida diet to rid yourself of the overgrowth of yeast. When I first had Candida and went on the Candida diet, I lost 20 pounds and felt the best I had ever felt in my life. The gas and intestinal pain I had been suffering from was completely gone.

Ghrelin as an Anti-Inflammatory Hormone

Ghrelin is the "hunger hormone", a peptide produced by ghrelin cells that are produced in the stomach, pancreas and in the gastrointestinal tract. Ghrelin duties are linked to a strategy your body uses to reduce inflammation, especially in your digestive tract. Ghrelin also helps protect your body from higher levels of the bacterial toxin known as lipopolysaccharide (LPS). Overweight people have higher levels of LPS, due to bacterial imbalance in the digestive tract. There is a blood test that reveals the higher levels in overweight people. Ghrelin helps clear your body of toxic LPS.

5

"BE A PEPPER" THE PH EATING PLAN

B e a Pepper, be a Tomato! Peppers and all of the vegetable family give us the best antioxidants and help boost our immune system. However they seem to be on the bottom of the list for popularity among most people but they are on the top of the list for helping to achieve an ideal pH.

pH means "potential of Hydrogen" measures our bodies to see if we are acidic, neutral or alkaline. Optimally, we want the fluids in our bodies to have a neutral pH level between 6.4 –7.0. Our pH can be measured from a blood test or from a urine test. I suggest shopping at your nearest health food store and purchase a box of pH strips for testing. It is very easy; you urinate on the pH strip first thing in the morning before you eat, drink or exercise then match the color of your strip to the color coded chart.

With the extreme toxicity that we live with today, finding a balance or neutral pH is not an easy task. I ask my clients to bring in their first morning urine on their first appointment with me. I have tested over 200 people and I have found only 4 people that had a neutral pH, and that is sad. I have even tested children and teenagers who were also all very acidic. A healthy pH has nothing to do with age. pH has much to do with how we live our lives, especially our diet. However, stress, alcohol, illnesses and toxic teeth will most certainly increase the probability of an acidic reading.

The color coded chart shows that pH ranges from 0 to 14. Battery acid is acidic and shows a pH reading of 1, the opposite of potassium which is highly alkaline and has a pH reading of 14. Since we are only concerned with body pH, the strips you buy will only cover a range from a 4.5 to an 8.0. The pH scale identifies the urine tested as anything under 6.4 as acidic and anything above 7.0 as alkaline.

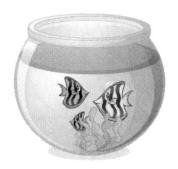

People with aquariums know that when the pH is off in the water, the fish will die. Any farmer can tell you that when the pH of the soil is too acidic or too alkaline, crops will become sickly and die. The same is true in the human body. An acidic pH creates a hostile internal environment, like a raging storm, making the body struggle to get the nutrients it needs. Urine is a liquid by-product of the body that is secreted by the kidneys. Why should we test our pH levels? Our bodies are made up of 50 to 60% water. pH effects our chemistry; it can promote health or sets the body up for disease. Urine pH readings are an indication of our body's health; it gives us a chance to make the changes we need to bring our bodies into superior health.

A cow that has a natural diet of grasses and other green leafy plants has a pH reading of the perfect 7 when measuring their digestive solution. This diet of green plants is a great source of Omega 3 fatty acid. A cow which is fed a diet consisting of mainly corn and grain will have a very acidic pH in their digestive solution. This is just one reason why organic milk is entirely different from unorganic milk.

Acidic pH

When your pH reading is low, 4.5 to 6.2, you are considered to be acidic, meaning your cells are deprived of oxygen and nutrients. An acidic pH can occur from, an acid diet, emotional stress, infections, surgeries, bad teeth, calcium deficiency in our bodies and much more. If the diet does not contain enough minerals, a buildup of acids will occur in the cells. An acidic body will show signs of infections, a loss of energy and disease at any age. An acidic body can start at any age, even in very young children. This is due to the nutrient deficient foods today, including antibiotics, growth hormones, GMO's, additives, preservatives, etc. An acidic pH lowers the immune system, making it unable to fight off toxicity and heal the body and make it much harder to lose weight, if at all. If your body is acidic, it becomes harder and harder for you to absorb nutrients. The key is to establish the proper acid/alkaline balance in your body. The more acidic you are, the worse you will most likely feel. Feeling lousy, pessimistic, angry, irritable, and fatigued are often symptoms of an acid system. Vitamin D is also directly required, along with the calcium to help the body absorb the calcium.

Too Alkaline

If the pH becomes too alkaline, (over 7.3), our cells become poisoned by their own toxic waste and start to die. This is called ammonia dumping, a sign that our bodies are so depleted from minerals that they are taking minerals out of our bones and organs just to survive. A pH over 8.0 is a serious danger signal, showing that the body has desperately recruited emergency supplies of ammonia as a last resort to buffer the extreme acid conditions of the body. This is most often due to a longstanding highly acid state which has depleted the body's mineral reserves, especially calcium. This is also why urine can have a distinctive smell of ammonia.

"Raise the Bar" Why is it so important to have good pH?

Remember, each 0.1 rise in pH means a 10-fold increase in oxygen! So if you started with a pH of 5.5 or below (the norm in the U.S.), and went to 7.0, you would have a 150-fold increase in tissue oxygen. Harmful virus and bacteria thrive in an acid (low-oxygen) rich environment. The neutral range gives oxygen to cells to help raise the mineral and vitamin levels in our body. By raising my own pH has boosted my immune system, keeping me very healthy. I have been exposed to many sick people, especially in the winter months, but have not caught any sicknesses in five years. pH is a great way to visually see your improvement. Don't get discouraged because if you carry lots of infections, especially in your teeth, your pH may not go up very much. This test will let you know that you still need to do more detoxing to become healthy.

"Give us this day our daily" Fruits and Vegetables?

The best way to start healing your body is to consume 70 percent of your daily food from the alkalizing side of the food chart. You will notice that your diet will contain many vegetables and some fruits. This will start to bring nutrition into your body to help fight off some of the toxicity build up. If you are starting from a diet of fast food, lunch meats, hot dogs, processed foods, white flour and white sugar, then you may experience detox symptoms. The alkalizing foods will start to eat up some of the toxicity, releasing in into your blood stream. This may cause symptoms such as fatigue, headaches, swelling and upset stomach. The good news is that within a few days to weeks your body will start to improve.

Many Americans often consume high-protein diets, which rapidly exhaust the body's mineral reserves. The kidneys, lungs and skin must work overtime to balance body pH toward the alkaline. Our bodies are so intelligent that if calcium, magnesium and potassium are not available when needed, it will borrow them from our bones and tissues. This is why you see older people slumped over, Osteoporosis, the weakening and deterioration of bones and muscles.

Bring up pH with Calcium

It is important for anyone over the age of 40 to add a calcium supplement to help bring up your pH. I recommend Coral Legend from Premier Research Labs. Coral Legend is a natural mineral powder made from coral harvested from the clear ocean bottom off the beautiful Japanese islands. The body must reduce any form of calcium into its ionic form in order to use it. Since Coral Legend contains calcium already in ionic form, the body can use the calcium immediately without having to break it down. Coral Legend is naturally balanced with ionic magnesium and many trace minerals for optimal mineral absorption. Unlike many other coral supplements on the market, this one has nothing added, and has no preservatives, fillers, or binders - Just pure marine-grade coral. By adding Premiers naturally made Vitamin D, along with the Coral legend you will have a guaranteed delivery system to ensure the proper absorption.

"Put a Tiger in Your Tank"

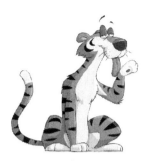

Choose the alkalizing fruits and veggies; they are a positive twofer, both alkalizing and fibrous! Since few people eat enough of the alkalinizing foods (fresh organic raw fruits and vegetables), and usually eat acidic foods (meats, dairy, sweets, soft drinks, and processed foods), I recommend that you start maximizing your nutrient intake by developing a balanced pH diet from the lists following. The pH diet shows us a list of foods that will help bring us into a healthy range. It is suggested that you eat 70% of your diet from the alkalizing chart and 30% from the acidic side. Make sure most of your diet is organic. Dumping more chemicals into your already toxic body is going to slow your healing and weight loss. Bring your pH into the neutral range of 6.4 to 7.0.

Alkalizing Foods
Alkalizing Vegetables

- Alfalfa
- Barley Grass
- Beets
- Broccoli
- Cabbage
- Carrot
- Cauliflower
- Celery
- Chard Greens
- Chlorella
- Collard Greens
- Cucumber
- Dandelions
- Eggplant

- Fermented Veggies
- Garlic
- Green Beans
- Green Peas
- Kale
- Kohlrabi
- Lettuce
- Mushrooms
- Mustard Greens
- Night Shades
- Onions
- Parsnips
- Peas
- Peppers

- Pumpkin
- Radishes
- Rutabaga
- Sea Veggies
- Spinach
- Spirulina
- Squash
- Sprouts
- Sweet Potatoes
- Tomatoes
- Watercress
- Wheat Grass
- Wild Greens

Alkalizing Asian Vegetables

- Daikon
- Dandelion Root
- Kombu
- Maitake
- Nori
- Reishi
- Shitake
- Umeboshi
- Wakame

Alkalizing Fruits

- Apple
- Apricot
- Avocado
- Banana
- Blueberries
- Blackberries
- Cantaloupe
- Cherries, sour
- Coconut, fresh
- Cranberries
- Currants
- Dates, dried
- Figs, dried
- Grapes NO (very toxic)
- Grapefruit
- Honeydew Melon
- Lemon
- Lime
- Muskmelons
- Nectarine
- Orange
- Peach
- Pear
- Plums
- Pineapple
- Raisins
- Raspberries
- Strawberries
- Tangerine
- Watermelon

Alkalizing Protein

- Almonds
- Chestnuts
- Millet
- Tempeh (fermented)
- Tofu (fermented)
- Chestnuts
- Millet
- Tempeh (fermented)
- Tofu (fermented)
- Whey Protein Powder
- Organic Chicken

Alkalizing Sweetener

- Stevia
- Coconut sugar
- Raw Honey

Alkalizing Other

- Alkaline Water
- Apple Cider Vinegar
- Bee Pollen
- Fresh Fruit Juice
- Green Juices
- Lecithin Granules
- Mineral Water
- Molasses, blackstrap
- Probiotic Cultures
- Soured Dairy Products
- Veggie Juices
- Green Juices
- Lecithin Granules
- Mineral Water
- Soured Dairy Products
- Veggie Juices

- Probiotic Cultures
- Coconut Water
- Almond Milk
- Quinoa
- Buckwheat
- Lentils
- Spelt
- White Beans
- Olives
- Avocado Oil
- Coconut Oil

Acidifying Other

- Black Beans
- Kidney Beans
- Chickpeas
- Millet
- Wheat
- White Flour
- Oats and Oatmeal
- Pinto Beans
- Red Beans
- Brown and white rice
- Soy Beans
- Soy Milk
- **Rye Bread**
- **All Pasta**

Acidifying Dairy

- Dairy
- Butter
- Cheese

- Cheese, Processed
- Ice Cream
- Ice Milk

Acidifying Nuts

- Cashews
- Legumes
- Peanut Butter (do not use any peanut products, mold)
- Peanuts
- Pecans
- Tahini
- Walnuts

Acidifying Animal Meats

- Bacon
- Beef
- Corned Beef
- Lamb
- Organ Meats
- Pork
- Rabbit
- Sausage
- Turkey
- Veal
- Venison

Acidifying Seafood

- Carp
- Clams
- Cod
- Fish
- Haddock
- Lobster

- Mussels
- Oyster
- Pike
- Salmon
- Sardines
- Scallops
- Shellfish
- Shrimp
- Tuna

Acidifying Oils

- Butter
- Canola Oil (do not use)
- Corn Oil   (do not use)
- Flax Oil
- Hemp Seed Oil
- Lard
- Olive Oil
- Safflower Oil
- Sesame Oil
- Sunflower Oil

Acidifying Sweeteners

- Carob
- Corn Syrup
- Sugar

Acidifying Others

- Catsup
- Cocoa
- Coffee
- Mustard
- Pepper
- Vinegar
- Iodized Salt

Acidifying Alcohol

- Beer
- Hard Liquor
- Spirits
- Wine

Acidifying Drugs

- Aspirin
- Chemicals
- Drugs, Medicinal
- Drugs, Psychedelic
- Herbicides
- Pesticides
- Tobacco

Acidifying Drinks

- Coca-Cola:
- Coffee

6

"NOT TIME TO MAKE THE DONUTS"
DIRTY DOZEN & CLEAN 15

It is almost impossible today to avoid toxicity, it is everywhere. By eating these poisonous pesticides that are regularly sprayed on our produce, we contaminate and increase the toxic load to our bodies. Chemical toxins affect everyone differently, but the one thing everyone has in common is that the toxins start to break down the body's immune system. With a compromised immune system, the body will no longer be able to protect itself from disease, infections and viruses. This is when most people will start to develop autoimmune diseases, and usually more than one at a time. Autoimmune diseases are when the immune system will start to attack itself causing: Lupus, Fibromyalgia, Celiac disease, Multiple Sclerosis, Psoriasis, Gluten Intolerance, Diabetes, Rheumatoid Arthritis, Grave's Disease, Hashimoto's Thyroid and Crohn's Disease just to name a few. Chemical pesticides found in foods have also been known to cause birth defects, cancer, damage to the nervous system and brain damage.

The dirty dozen are the highest contaminated fruits and vegetables with pesticides. It is important to become educated on what foods you need to buy Organic and which ones are less toxic that you can purchase without the Organic label. The best and safest way to eat without toxicity is to grow your own food or purchase from a local farmer, whom you trust, who does not spray with pesticides. The Environmental Working Group has released a list of the "Dirty

Dozen, veggies and fruits you should buy organic, and the "Clean Fifteen" fruits and vegetables that can be bought from conventional farming.

The Clean Fifteen are the safer fruits and vegetables to add to your diet. You will notice that most of them have a thicker skin, protecting them from heavy pesticide use. Always make sure to wash your vegetables; Premiers Limonene and Polar Mins are two of my personal favorites from PRL. You will be amazed at what comes off the vegetables and fruits when you wash them.

The EPA defines pesticides as "any agent used to kill or control undesired insects, weeds, rodents, fungi, bacteria, or other organisms. Herbicides control weeds and fungicides control fungi, mold and mildew. Herbicides are the most widely used type of pesticide in agriculture, although pest problems and their management vary widely throughout the country, depending on climate, soil types and other factors."

Strawberries are one of the most toxic sprayed fruits, using the largest amount of chemicals. Peaches and Nectarines use 45 different chemicals, bell peppers 39, apples 36, grapes 35, tomatoes 30, and celery 29. Spinach, kale and collard greens are also very toxic, and potatoes are grown in the ground, treated with chemicals first so it can grow right into the potato.

Try to eat one cup of cruciferous vegetables including cabbage, broccoli, collards, kale or brussel sprouts daily. Consume fresh homemade vegetable juice, eat berries and citrus fruits for bioflavonoids, eat celery to aid in urine flow, turmeric and curry for anti-inflammatory, and lots of dark green leafy vegetables.

The Clean 15

On a budget, choose these conventionally.
(Listed from lowest pesticide content)

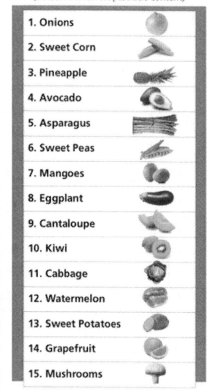

1. Onions
2. Sweet Corn
3. Pineapple
4. Avocado
5. Asparagus
6. Sweet Peas
7. Mangoes
8. Eggplant
9. Cantaloupe
10. Kiwi
11. Cabbage
12. Watermelon
13. Sweet Potatoes
14. Grapefruit
15. Mushrooms

The Dirty Dozen

Always buy these organic.
(Listed from highest pesticide content to least)

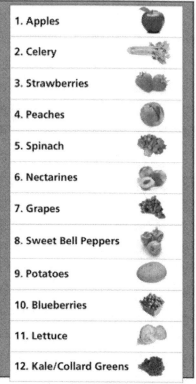

1. Apples
2. Celery
3. Strawberries
4. Peaches
5. Spinach
6. Nectarines
7. Grapes
8. Sweet Bell Peppers
9. Potatoes
10. Blueberries
11. Lettuce
12. Kale/Collard Greens

Source: Environmental Working Group 2011

7

"SNAP, CRACKLE, FLOP" ENERGY & ADRENALS

In my practice I have noticed that almost every client I see complains of low energy. It is not just older folks; I also see kids, teens and younger people that should not be energy deficient. Loss of energy comes from all types of stress; physical, mental and emotional stress. The immune system starts off strong when we are young, and the older we get we are exposed to toxins in the air, the water we drink, the sleep we do not get enough of, and the stress from, work, relationships and family. The food we eat also puts stress on our bodies such as; fast food, microwave food, processed foods, foods with antibiotics and hormones, and the list goes on and on. This stress will weaken our immune system and when we add mental, emotional and physical stress on top of it we get adrenal fatigue/burnout.

"For fast-Acting Relief Try Slowing Down."

Many of the people that I treated for adrenal fatigue had a "Type A" personality. They can be seen as very competitive, over achievers, workaholics, or adult children of alcoholics. This personality type can be loud, extraverts, aggressive, impatient, talk over others, walk and talk at a rapid pace, or are always engaged in an activity. They are also the ones you see at the gym working out for 2 hours or more. I know this type of personality quite well, since I am one of them and so are most of my friends and co-workers. Over the years, this type of extra stress that most "Type A" people experience takes a toll on one's health and lifestyle. We push, pull, and become work horses, many of us workaholics craving and running on adrenalin, or the drug norepinephrine, subsequently causing adrenal fatigue.

"Burn Baby Burn" Adrenal Fatigue/Burnout

I developed adrenal fatigue. For an entire year I was going from one medical doctor to the next with no avail. It is so frustrating to have no energy and have no one that is able to help you. The doctors told me there was nothing wrong with me. They did offer me antidepressants...Wth! Doc...I am not depressed, I do not have enough energy to get out of bed, or go to work. I was 51 years old and still having monthly periods. I had severe symptoms; <u>irregular heartbeats, vertigo, weak, shaky, throbbing in thyroid, insomnia, pain in joints and muscles, toe and finger nails ridges, hair loss, sore throat, constant cold symptoms, low body temp, low pulse, low blood pressure, cold all the time, loss of memory and concentration.</u> In addition to these, some people may have depression, pain in the low back area and perhaps excessive thirst or craving for sweet and salty foods. A doc did put me on thyroid meds for a while but there was no change. I also put on 50 pounds while I had adrenal fatigue. If you have adrenal fatigue there is NO WAY YOU WILL LOSE WEIGHT!

The adrenal glands are disc-shaped glands that sit on top of each kidney. The adrenals secrete hormones that prepare our bodies for stress, producing adrenalin or epinephrine, norepinephrine, cortisol, estrogens, testosterone, progesterone, DHEA and pregnenolone. Wow powerful little buggers. These hormones help us to promote energy production, raise blood pressure and regulate glucose in the blood. Basically every time you have a stress reaction, an adrenaline rush, panic attack or feeling stressed or anxious, your body secretes the hormone cortisol. The following is a list of disorders caused from too much cortisol:

Abdominal obesity (belly fat)
High blood sugar (adrenal diabetes)
Muscle wasting
Bone loss
Immune shutdown
Thin wrinkled skin
Fluid retention Hypertension

There are a couple of tests that can determine if you have Adrenal fatigue. The first is called the Ragland test. A practitioner will take your blood pressure while lying down and then again when you stand up. Your blood pressure should go up when you stand up. Mine went down, and so will yours if you have adrenal fatigue. I remember being dizzy and shaky when I stood up. Another test I did by myself at home is to shine a flashlight in one of your eyes. Look in the mirror to see if the pupil, the black part, constricts quickly. Mine remained large. If the pupil does not constrict this is another sign of adrenal fatigue. Another sign is that no matter how much sleep you get, you are always tired or exhausted. I took a saliva hormone test which showed that my cortisol levels were very low. You can also get a hair analysis which can show cortisol levels and different metals that are high in the body. This was my official confirmation that I had adrenal fatigue. At least I had a name for what I was suffering from. It felt so good to know I was not crazy and really was sick.

"Clean up on Isle 3"

Your clean-up starts with rest, relaxation and rejuvenation. Now if you are that Type A personality, this is not going to be easy. You will still be pushing and making excuses like "I have to do the laundry, cut the grass, etc." The physical exertion has to stop here, along with worrying about how you will get things done. It's not easy, but you have to rest. You will make things worse, get even dizzier, and start to run yourself into the ground.

The rejuvenation will start with the removal of toxicity from your body and the nourishment your body needs such as good foods and the proper supplements to treat your deficiencies. I highly suggest buying a juicer and start to make your own juice with mostly vegetable and some fruit. (More on Juicing in Chapter 17)

A diet high in carbohydrates and low in protein will add more stress on the adrenals. Also, not consuming enough good quality water is essential for the bodies function. Many diets are low in nutrients, so a person with adrenal issues will need to enrich their bodies with Premiers vitamin E (Deltinol), Premier's AdrenaVen is a must, in addition to RenaVen and a complex B vitamin, Premiers

Max B. Many people with Adrenal issues suffer with digestive issues and are unable to eliminate daily. Remember our immune system is in our gut, so if the body is unable to get rid of the poisons and toxins in our body, they are reabsorbed into the body. You will need Premiers HCL, Hydrochloric Acid at a very minimum to help digest your food. If your diet has been extremely poor, I would suggest looking into colon hydrotherapy. This has been a staple in my life for twenty years and has helped me out tremendously. A QRA appointment will be necessary to complete your recovery and re-nourish the entire body. Then the adrenals begin to function normally and one's energy will return. (More on QRA in Chapter 13)

Another issue I had which contributed to my adrenal fatigue was my toxic teeth; the mercury and infections in my root canals. (more on this in Chapter 11) I still had a return of my headaches and vertigo until the last tooth was removed. What is so amazing is that I was dizzy every day for six weeks in 2014, and the very day my last root canal tooth was removed, my vertigo disappears and has never returned. It is a must to make an appointment with a holistic dentist that can run tests to see if you will need repairs or removals. I can't tell you how important this is.

"Worry Bankrupts Our Spirit, So Relax"
Ways to Reduce High Stress

1. Use a cortisol reducing supplement: There are a variety of herbs to reduce cortisol at peak times. Some of my favorites include: Premiers Tranquinol and Premiers Melatonin.
2. Make sure you get to bed on time. The best time is 10:00pm, and you should try and get at least 8 hours of sleep. If you have adrenal fatigue you are probably getting this much sleep and also taking naps. That is ok for now. Give in to your body and get the rest you need. Some people will not be able to sleep, which is ironic when you are exhausted, so you will need to make sure you are on the proper supplements to help nourish your adrenals.

3. Eat at regular intervals throughout the day. You will need to avoid skipping meals so you will not create a cortisol release.
4. Eliminate all sodas, coffee, energy drinks and replace them with home-made green tea, lots of filtered water and the most important Premiers Max B. Make sure to detox slowly off all caffeine beverages.
5. Eliminate all junk food, fast food, and limit your simple carbohydrates including grains and breads. Carbohydrates create cortisol release in response to the elevated insulin levels. Eat more fruits and vegetables. Eat a balanced diet of protein, veggies, fruits, and good quality fats.
6. Reduce your stress by learning relaxation techniques: meditation, Reiki, hypnosis and a lot of deep breathing. Get a massage and take a yoga class. Everything in your life must be centered on relaxation. (Read more about relaxation techniques in Chapter 19)
7. Do not exercise, at first not even walking. Exercise causes the body to release cortisol. Remember we need to conserve energy now, not exert it.

Cortisol is a steroid hormone that is produced in the cortex of the adrenal glands. Cortisol is released with a peak secretion in the early morning, and then it tapers out in the late afternoon and evening for people that do not have adrenal fatigue. If you have adrenal fatigue, your peaks and valleys will be erratic, spiking in the evening instead of going down. Many people with adrenal issues are unable to sleep at night due to these spikes. I had trouble going to sleep because my cortisol would rise up at night. So you need sleep and can't get it!

8

"THE GOOD, BAD AND UGLY" HORMONE BALANCE

H ormone balance is not easy and many women are affected by nasty symptoms from an early age with the onset of our periods; PMS, painful cramps, and irritability. It doesn't end there, we are blessed even more, when we stop our periods suffering with hormone imbalance that comes with menopause. With a lifetime of toxicity adding to our already mineral and vitamin deficient bodies, we are a hot mess. Most of us suffer horribly with hot flashes and night sweats, and in this state we start to really pack on the pounds. On the next page you will see a chart that identifies all of the hormones in our body. Both men and women have these hormones, so you will see how important each one is and what their jobs are. This is why it is so hard to get the right mix of hormones to get us back on track. Usually, if you are not already overweight from all the other issues in this book, you will gain most of your weight in the late forties/ early fifties. Hormone imbalance also affects men in their late forties and they will most likely need Premiers Testosterone or ProstaVen.

Thyroid

The thyroid is one of the most challenging hormones to balance and the estimate is that 1 out of every 5 Americans have a thyroid issue. When the thyroid is not producing the right amount of hormones, many will feel depressed, have low energy, cold hands and feet, and gain weight. Since I have seen over 200 people in my practice, I've found that 1 out of every 2 women tested have a thyroid issue. Of course most of my practice consists of women age 45 -55. The QRA testing will test all of the hormonal areas. Some women may only need one supplement and others may need a combination of several to stop the menopause symptoms. The thyroid is addressed separately. Remember that QRA will find a malfunctioning thyroid issue many years before a doctor can find it in a blood test. When a doc finds it, the thyroid has usually deteriorated to an exhausted state. It can still be brought back to life with the proper nutrition, nutritional supplements and detoxing. The most important supplements for your thyroid are going to be Premiers Xenostat, Thyroven and Green tea. Make sure to get your thyroid tested to determine which supplements are best to use to bring you and your thyroid back to life. Eating radishes has been known to help balance out your thyroid, so pack them into your salads or even better, juice them.

Moans, Groans, Stones, and Bones
If you have any of the symptoms below you may
have a hormone imbalance:

Loss of energy	Don't quite feel normal
Lazy, Lethargic	Feel old
Tired all the time	Can't concentrate
Chronic fatigue	Depression
Just don't feel well	Osteoporosis and Osteopenia

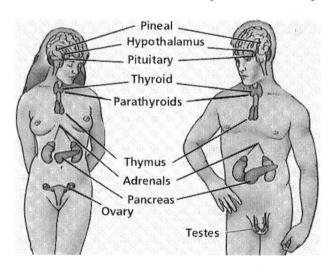

Pineal
Hypothalamus
Pituitary
Thyroid
Parathyroids

Thymus
Adrenals
Pancreas
Ovary

Testes

Bones hurt: legs and arms

Wake up in middle of night

Trouble getting to sleep

Tired during the day

Irritable and cranky

Forget simple things

Gastric acid reflux

Heartburn; GERD

Decrease in sex drive

Thinning hair

Kidney stones

High Blood Pressure

Recurrent Headaches

Heart Palpitations (arrhythmias)

Estrogens are produced in the ovaries, placenta, liver, adrenals, fat and cells. Their function is for female development, menstruation, pregnancy, and antiaging.

Pregnenolone is produced in the adrenals. It is responsible for memory and stress resistance.

Cortisol is produced in the adrenals. It is responsible for stress, energy production, mood stability and inflammatory responses.

Vitamin D is produced in the skin, liver and kidneys. It is responsible for muscle, bone and heart health, immunity, cell communication and brain development.

Human Growth Hormone (HGH) is produced in the placenta. It promotes growth in children and adolescents and helps regulate body composition, tissue growth and metabolism in adults.

Melatonin is produced in the pineal gland. It helps promote sleep, supports brain health, heart health, and immune system.

Glucagon is produced in the pancreas. It signals glucose to be transferred to the blood into your cells for energy usage and fat body regulation. It also signals the liver to release glucose into your blood.

Parathyroid Hormone is produced in the parathyroid gland. It controls the amount of calcium in your blood and bones.

Adrenalin is produced in the adrenals. It regulates heart rate, releases glucose and dilates blood vessels.

Thyroid hormone is produced in the thyroid gland. It is responsible for organ development and metabolism.

Progesterone is produced in the ovaries, placenta and the Central Nervous System (CNS.) It is responsible for breast development, female sexual development, menstruation, and pregnancy.

Testosterone is produced in the testes and ovaries. They are responsible for male sexual development, sex drive, sperm production and bone and muscle mass.

DHEA is produced in the adrenals and brain. They are responsible for lean body mass, heart health, resistance to stress, and lean body mass.

Ghrelin is produced in the stomach and pancreas. Its job is for fat regulation and stimulates hunger. Ghrelin is a little gremlin in your stomach that makes you want to tear up some food. Just remember, *"Don't Feed Them after Midnight,"* this little hunger hormone sends messages and travels to your brain and impacts your desire to eat. If you have major food cravings you most likely have a malfunctioning ghrelin. The more you crave sugar, high calorie foods and carbohydrates the greater your problem. It can also cause a subconscious desire to binge eating or stuffing yourself to give you a pleasurable feeling of fullness or satisfaction. Ghrelin activation is vital to maintain your blood sugar during calorie restriction or starvation.

Make sure you stop eating 3 to 4 hours before you go to bed. You do not want your body digesting food as you start to go to bed. Digestion is a major problem which keeps people up at night, unable to get or stay asleep.

Leptin is produced in the fat cells. It controls fat regulation. Most people that are overweight suffer from a leptin resistance, where it perceives a false state of starvation. This is very important because it activates the ghrelin, even if we are full, and confuses our metabolism.

9

"MUNCH A BUNCH OF" SUPPLEMENTS

The saddest part of my practice is the thousands of supplements people bring in that I have used the QRA testing technique and have found them to be inferior for one of the many reasons listed below. This is why I choose and recommend that you purchase your supplements from Premier Research Labs. The following are guidelines Premier uses with every supplement they sell:

1. No magnesium stearate, undesirable oil that can suppress the immune system.
2. No animal glandular with toxic tagalongs and unwanted animal hormones.
3. No tablets with toxic tagalong binders and fillers.
4. No excipients - Excipients are highly questionable (often problematic) fillers and binders which are commonly added to nutritional products.
5. Protect ingredients using Violite® bottles or glass. Violite® is PRL's patent-pending, dark violet-colored, PET plastic bottle that is engineered to block the light frequencies from 450-720 nanometers, which create radiation damage to ingredients.
6. PRL conducts scientific laboratory testing of every incoming container of raw material and all finished products. PRL Uses high performance Crystal Spectroscopy to assure the potency and reliability of every ingredient and to scan for contaminants that are typically in many

other products such as radiation, heavy metals, pesticides and excess moisture.

7. Premier uses vegetable capsules instead of capsules made from animal products. They use no damaging heat or pressure, no degrading of nutrients, no rancid oil by-products, no toxic glues, binders or lubricants. The veggie caps dissolve easily in the stomach.

8. Premiers vitamins and supplements are made from all live sources, mostly live plants and a few from live animals done humanely and never harming the animal in any way. "So who you gonna call, synthetic busters." Premier Research Labs. 800-325-7734.

There are other companies that sell supplements that make a good product, but you will have to do your research to find them. Make sure to check the products with the process listed on the previous page. If you buy un-organic products you are most likely putting more toxins in your body, and that "*does not do a body good.*"

Skip the Synthetic Cesspool/ Fake Supplements

Synthetic vitamins lack the energy from the source needed to unlock the vitamin's potential. As a result, the body must detoxify itself of these "toxins" through the liver and kidneys. Thus, any positive benefits from vitamin supplementation are lost. Most synthetic vitamins like A, B, C D & E are "created" in labs.

1. Most B vitamins are synthesized from coal tar, acetonitrile with ammonia, hydrochloric acid; can you believe it? If you are taking this, you will notice that your urine is a real dark orange color from the tar, you will see it listed as thiamin mononitrate or thiamin HCL on the label. Make sure to check labels.

2. Most ascorbic acid or synthetic vitamin C is made by fermenting corn sugar into sorbitol, hydrogenation and adding acetone (i.e. nail polish remover).

3. Vitamin D3 is made from Dristol which is irradiating fungus and plant matter.
4. Vitamin A is made from benzene, methanol, petroleum esters and refined oils.
5. Synthetic form of vitamin E- dl-alpha tocopherol, dl-alpha tocopherol acetate or succinate.

Almost all vitamin C sold in the United States is made in China. Since the United States does not require country-of-origin labels for any of our drugs, foods or supplements, there is no telling where the vitamin you are taking came from. Don't be fooled, read the label. If it does not say "naturally occurring" and list the name of the food source, then let the buyer beware that they are synthetic. If a food is grown in China organically, there is no testing or limitation on how many heavy metals, BPA, or synthetic chemicals are contained in their so called organic product.

"Health doesn't happen by accident, it happens on Purpose"

Are you willing to do anything to restore your body to health? Will you find the energy, time and money to heal yourself? Are you worth it? YES!

How Long Will It Take?

How much abuse has your body been through and for how long? Healing takes as long as you dedicate your time and energy to your program. It's like peeling an onion: We start with the nutrients that your body has picked, and then move to detox all of the interference fields that have been affected though our ABUSE.

Definition of Health:

"Eat Well, Move Well, Think Well"

Change your diet and bring supplements with nutrition back into the body. Take a walk or stretch out with yoga. Work on clearing out the negativity and be present and positive.

"Don't Leave Home Without Them"

My healing started when I took Premier's supplements. I was so very sick so I needed a large quantity of supplements. One thing to remember is that most doses of just one supplement may require you to take six a day. Taking supplements are nutrients that come alive in the body and start to give weak and sick organs the nutrients they need to actually feed them and heal them. Most of us have taken some sort of medication in our lifetime so we know you take just one pill at a time. Once you start a medication, you will remain on it for the rest of your life. Medications are also acidic, and we know now from the previous chapter how it can cause disease if we stay acidic. Medications can save lives, such as an antibiotic in life threating situation like Ebola. However, have you ever heard of someone healing from a medication? Of course not! They are intended to bring down numbers such as diabetes and cholesterol. So many prescriptions are unnecessary as they are so over prescribed. God gave us an immune system, so let's use it! We can build back up what we have torn down, but it is going to take time. It has taken you a lifetime to become sick and fat, so it may take months or longer for you to heal. I can tell you after only a couple weeks, I felt so much better after detoxing and taking supplements from Premier. Below are my favorites and a must for someone that is sick. Play it safe…buy real food supplements.

RenaVen

This premier quality, broad-spectrum formula offers effective support for detoxification and optimal kidney health. The kidney is one of the most important organs because it is constantly filtering and detoxifying all of the toxins we take in. RenaVen™features three key botanical blends: Agari-Pro™, an Agaricus bisporus extract (175 mg/capsule) and Agari-Plex Detox™, the perfect support blend. You must strengthen the kidney since you will be detoxing so many toxins through the kidneys and out of your body.

HCL

HCL is the most important supplement, and should be a household name, that needs to be a staple in your diet. HCL puts hydrochloric acid back into our stomach to enable us to digest food as our bodies were intended to. HCL contains 100% natural-source betaine hydrochloride from beets, created to assist in the digestion and absorption of nutrients, especially protein, vitamin B12, calcium, iron and other minerals. As we age, our production of HCL starts to diminish, which is why so many of us turn 40 and all of a sudden suffer from gas, bloating, GERD, IBS, and reflux.

I have seen a people come into my office wondering why they can't seem to handle that chili hot dog anymore. Really! Some go to great lengths to continue to eat that hot dog such as getting a prescription from their doctors. By taking that prescription, it will take the acid out of the stomach so there are no symptoms from that hot dog. Symptoms are a wakeup call, telling us that something is wrong. Instead of eating the hot dog, maybe it is time to eat different foods. When you take HCL, it puts hydrochloric acid back into your stomach, making it easier to digest food. Doesn't that make more sense?

Max B

Max B is my favorite and I take it every day. Many of our customers can feel instant energy from our Max B. The liquid form ensures quick delivery and absorption. Our cells prefer Max B's live source, high energy, end-chain vitamin B forms, over common synthetic (coal tar-derived) sources. This B vitamin-rich formula offers advanced support for the liver, energy, immune system, adrenals and mood balance. Carbohydrates can cause vitamin B deficiencies. Problems associated with B vitamin deficiencies include depression, memory loss, heart disease, insomnia, cataracts, atherosclerosis, fatigue, muscle cramps, allergies and GI symptoms to name just a few.

AdrenaVen

This product is a must for those with adrenal fatigue. AdrenaVen™ is a premier-quality master formula designed to support healthy adrenal glands, which produce hormones for your organs to function. It features prickly pear, antioxidant qualities and it is also rich in Vitamin C.

WHY CAN'T I LOSE WEIGHT? TOXINS

Green Tea ND

Green Tea ND is one of my favorites to help bring energy and healing for those who suffer from a dysfunctional thyroid or just a loss of energy. Green tea leaves are high in polyphenols, which boost the metabolism and help with anti-aging, digestive function, joint flexibility, healthy immune response and rejuvenation support.

Adaptogen-R3

Adaptogens are certain herbs particularly helpful in restoring and maintaining positive homeostasis, the body's natural ability to balance internal and external stress. Adaptogen-R3 is very helpful in supporting hormone balance, hot flashes, weight gain and night sweats. Adaptogen-R3™ contains Nopal cactus, Fo Ti, Rhodiola Rosea and Ecklonia Cava, an invigorating formula that promotes the entire adaptogenic process, including whole body rejuvenation.

Immuno-ND

Immuno-ND™ is a live-source, probiotic-derived concentrate that provides premier detoxification and immune system support. Immuno-ND™ uses bark from the Pau d'Arco tree. We highly recommend Immuno-ND for individuals with an imbalanced lymphatic system, commonly present with those who have a diet high in cooked grains and frequent alcoholic beverage consumption. Immuno-ND is helpful in opening up the lymph nodes to get rid of toxins and infection.

UltraPollen

UltraPollen™ is made from premier quality, multiple flower pollen extracts (300 mg/cap) that are 100% allergen and pesticide free (mold spore removed). This premier formula delivers extraordinary flower pollen-based support for health and wellness. UltraPollen is our first choice for those who want to achieve hormone balance. Symptoms of hormone imbalance include a diet high in refined food and a body burden of toxic pesticides/plastic residues.

OsteoVen

OsteoVen is our first choice for those with bone issues. OsteoVen™ is a comprehensive formula that provides premier quality support for healthy bones, joint function and connective tissue. One of its key ingredients is a type of yucca named Adam's Needle. Symptoms of poor bone and joint health include dental issues, poor digestion and side effects caused by prescription drugs.

Cardio-ND

Cardio ND delivers comprehensive support for the cardiovascular system. This is one of our most popular practitioner formulas for cardiovascular support. One of the main ingredients is Hawthorn Berry, which has been used for centuries in Europe to strengthen the heart and treat angina.

Coral Legend

Coral Legend is one of our most popular supplements because many of our supplements cannot be absorbed in the body without calcium. Coral Legend provides 100% pure Sango marine coral powder (no fillers or additives such as ground sand), delivering premier calcium and magnesium minerals with an impressive 2:1 ratio for superb mineral support. This powder concentrate is a top seller due to its legendary mineral support for the bones, joints and in promoting a healthy alkaline pH for whole body health and vitality.

Aloe Pro

This organic aloe is not loaded with undesirable preservatives such as sodium benzoate. Our pure aloe liquid provides the complete array of aloe's inherent beneficial properties and is unheated and completely intact. Aloe is high in vitamins, minerals, amino acids and fatty acids. It is usually mixed with Coral Legend and D3 for the perfect trio.

D3

A one-of-a-kind, live-source vitamin D3 delivers cardiovascular and immune system support. Vitamin D3 also aids in calcium absorption for healthy bones and teeth. Recent studies propose ideal vitamin D3 intake should be 2000 IU or more daily (a recommendation our serum meets in just one drop). Our D3 is made with extra virgin olive oil.

EFA

Our distinctive oil blend, which includes the use of flaxseed oil, is a premier quality life-essential fatty acid formula for optimal brain and body support, featuring an ideal blend of GLA (gamma linolenic acid) and Omega 3, 6 and 9 essential fatty acids. Premier EFA Oil Blend is comprised of cold-pressed, premier, unrefined oils that are nitrogen-flushed to protect freshness. This blend has a full-bodied gourmet taste that is delicious mixed in food or drinks.

DHA

DHA is an essential plant-source that is derived from non-GMO micro-algae instead of fish, making it suitable for everyone including vegetarians and vegans. Feed your brain with plant-source DHA (docosahexaenoic acid), a key Omega-3 fatty acid, important for the brain, nervous system, eyes and cardio-vascular health.

43 Uses for Premiers Coconut Oil

1. Eat a spoonful to get your daily oil, immune and energy boost.
2. Use to condition your wooden cutting boards.
3. Use as a super conditioner on your hair (apply to dry hair, leave in as long as possible and then shampoo as normal).
4. Use as a styling agent if you have really dry hair. Just rub a tiny bit on your palms and apply to your hair and style as normal.
5. Lip moisturizer.
6. Add a spoonful to your dog or cat's food, or give by spoon. Mine love it.
7. As a cooking and baking oil.
8. Use it for oil pulling (swish around your mouth to fight infection in mouth)
9. Use to oil your pans and baking dishes instead of pan spray.
10. Mix a tiny dab with baking soda for a natural deodorant.

11. Use coconut oil instead of shaving cream.
12. Use as a daily body moisturizer, add a scent.
13. Use as a makeup remover.
14. Use it to help sooth chicken pox, shingles, or other rashes or skin irritations.
15. Use it to treat athlete's food, ringworm, or other fungal or yeast infections.
16. Take a spoonful with your vitamins to help improve absorption.
17. Spread a thin layer on cuts or burns to speed up healing.
18. Take up to 5 spoonful's per day for improved thyroid function.
19. Add a spoonful to your smoothies for extra nutrition and flavor.
20. Use on the delicate tissue around your eyes to help prevent wrinkles and sagging.
21. Use as the base for homemade toothpaste.
22. Use in place of massage oil.
23. Use on your baby's diaper rash or cradle cap.
24. For nursing mothers, use coconut oil on your nipples to prevent cracking and irritation.
25. For nursing mothers, consuming coconut oil can help increase your milk flow.
26. Women can use vaginally to relieve yeast infections, dryness, and/or discomfort.
27. Eat a spoonful with each meal to improve digestion.
28. Helps soothe and heal hemorrhoids.
29. Mix with peppermint, eucalyptus, and rosemary for homemade vapor rub.
30. Mixed with tea tree, peppermint, lemon balm, rosemary, makes an excellent insect repellant.
31. Use to help detox the body, during a cleanse.
32. Apply to bee stings or bug bites to soothe and heal.
33. Use as a metal polish, but always test a small area first.
34. Use as a leather moisturizer. (test a small area first)
35. Season your cast iron pans.

36. Remove gum from your hair.
37. Take a spoonful to help with heartburn, acid reflux, or indigestion.
38. Use as a natural sunscreen. Limit your time in the sun, don't overdo it.
39. Mix with a tiny bit of fresh lemon juice and use as a furniture polish. (always test a small area first!)
40. Moisturize cracked or rough heals. (use at night, put socks on, wake up smooth)
41. Massage into your nails and cuticles to help strengthen them.
42. Take a couple spoonful's every day to help overall immune function.
43. Mix with organic sugar for a homemade body scrub.

10

"NOTHING COMES BETWEEN ME AND MY GENES"

Have you ever seen a woman, carrying a newborn baby, and she looks like she was never pregnant? Do you know someone, male or female, who fit in the same clothes they did when they were in high school?...and you hate them. You wonder why they never gain weight. Genetics are very strong and if you come from thin you will most likely stay thin. Doesn't seem fair, but if they ever do stem cell skinny genes I will be the first in line.

"Play Ball"

Strike one – You have one overweight parent. I am not talking about overweight parents as adults because half the population is there. I am talking about large as a child. My dad was also large as a child, having to wear husky clothes.

Strike two – You are female. Women have a higher percentage of body fat than men. Men have more muscle making their metabolism more efficient. Muscle burns more fat even while a person is at their resting metabolic rate.

Strike three - You are over the age of 50!

You're not out you just need to keep your eye on the ball.

"Fat is as Fat Does" Fat Kids Beware

Everyone is born with a certain number of fat cells. As an adult we can have between 10 and 30 billion fat cells. So if we pig out and gain weight when we are young, the fat cells start adding up, increasing the amount of fat cells. So a young person or child that is overweight as a child will have more fat cells then someone that was not overweight, usually twice the amount. The good news is you can lose them while you are still a child. Unfortunately, by the time we reach 20 we cannot lose fat cells, so you are stuck with the increased amount.

But get this...you can still increase the amount of fat cells; the more you eat and gain, those fat cells keep expanding and if they get big enough they start to divide and create more cells. Well that's not fair! Then as we age our fat cells start to die off, well that sounds good right? No as they die off they regenerate, keeping that dreaded number of fat cells the same. The more fat cells we have, the harder it is to lose weight. It's ok...we can still lose weight by reducing the amount of fat out of the cell, making us a mean, lean machine! It may be too late for us to reduce the amount of fat cells, but if you have small children, make sure they do not become overweight during childhood.

Another problem is many people that are dieting do not include good fats in their diet. Our fat cells need good fat. So if you don't feed your fat, your body will send out a message, "FEED ME." If you don't...what do you think you will start to crave? FAT and most likely the wrong kind, *"Back away from the fries!"*

So genes can't be changed, but they can be turned on with exercise. If you are the kind of person that eats a donut and it goes right to your butt, then exercise is now your new best friend. The phenomenon is called epigenetics, DNA methylation. DNA is in every cell and has our own little blueprint of who we are, or who are parents were. So to keep it simple, methyl groups can control if the gene is active or inactive. So guess what? Exercise puts your gene in overdrive....it revs up those fat genes.

"Exercise, You Don't Have Time Not To"

New research from Lund University in Sweden, reported in *PLoS Genetics* June 27, 2013, described for the first time what happens in fat cells when we exercise. They studied the methyl groups in fat cells of 23 overweight and inactive men around 35 years old. These men exercised twice a week for six months doing either a spin class or aerobics class. What they found was that exercise altered the methylation pattern in 7,000 out of 480,000 genes that were observed. It changed the pattern of fat storage in the genes. Another study compared the gene alteration from a group that burned off 400 calories. One group burned it with an intense workout, the other group with a low impact workout. What they found was intensity does matter. The group that worded out harder had more change to their fat in their gene storage. It also showed that by just doing one workout can also affect your gene mutation.

"Thing 1, Thing 2"

There have been a lot of studies done with twins that support the genetic weight factor. "About 50 percent of adult-onset weight change remains genetic," principal investigator James C. Romeis, a professor of health services research, said in a prepared statement. He studied almost 4,000 sets of male twins who served in the military during the Vietnam War. The study revealed that genes account for 50 percent of the change in body mass index and the other 50 percent is due to diet and exercise. Another study of 311 pairs of twins who had been raised apart and 362 pairs who had been raised together showed the results of obesity between the two had little or no influence on obesity, showing environment was not much of a factor.

In the Journal of Science and the Journal of Clinical Investigation, researchers describe new genetic factors that help to describe weight gain in people. Researcher at the Boston Children's Hospital found a rare genetic mutation that prevented mice from burning off fat calories. The mutation, Mrap2gene, showed that they fed a group of mice with this mutated gene less food and they still gained weight. When they fed the mice the same amount of calories as the group with no mutation, they noticed the mice continued to gain weight. The control group did not gain weight like the mutated mice. They also found the same gene was mutated in a group of obese people. The studies found that weight gain is a combination of different metabolic processes, from brain systems that regulate appetite to enzymes that control how calories are turned from food into either energy or fat.

The scientists found a similar pattern among a group of 500 obese people; they detected four mutations in the human version of Mrap2, and each of the obese individuals possessed only one bad version of the gene.

<u>Leptin:</u> is known as the "obesity hormone." Leptin is made by fat cells and acts as a thermostat for the body's energy needs. Each person has his own leptin threshold; if leptin levels fall to a lower level, the brain understands that

the body is starving, and needs more food. If leptin levels are maintained or surge above that amount, the brain knows that it doesn't need to take in more food. However if a person is leptin-resistant people do not get the signal to stop eating.

Ghrelin: This gene makes an appetite hormone that can make foods look more desirable especially high-calorie ones, by influencing the brain's reward system. Some studies have found that people who are sleep deprived have increased ghrelin levels, which may explain why lack of sleep can contribute to weight gain.

"Be All You Can Be"

If you inherited a slow metabolism, then you will have to learn how to rev up your metabolism. Exercise is going to be the best way for you to do this. I recommend that you start off by walking. Once you start walking you will need to start increasing your pace with short bursts of quick walking. You will need to take it easy if you are just starting to exercise, have adrenal fatigue or are considered to be in bad health. Always consult your physician before starting an exercise program. Again, if you are just starting to detox, you will need to take it easy and just walk or practice yoga and meditation.

We already know the benefits of exercise; controls weight, combats disease, gives us energy, improves our mood and can even help us to sleep better. If you are in good health, I recommend you join a gym and start to build yourself up to a rigorous health program. Weight lifting is going to be a positive factor in building muscle to help rev up your metabolism and help your body to burn off the fat and build muscle.

11

"TAKING AIM AGAINST CAVITIES" TOXIC TEETH

In the United States, people are exposed to mercury from three major sources; fish and shellfish (methylmercury/organic), vaccines (ethylmercury), and dental amalgams (elemental mercury in the form of mercury vapor). All forms of mercury are known to be dangerous and can cause damage to our bodies.

As a kid, I ate a whole lot of sugar candy and chewed a ton of sugar gum. When I was sixteen I had 17 cavities. So I was drilled and filled and also had my wisdom teeth pulled. I hated the dentist from a very young age. When I turned 40, I started getting root canals as a final attempt to save my teeth. By 50 I was sick.

Part of my training with Premier is that we get educated with an array of different toxins that can affect a person's health. Dr. Gene Sambataro, a holistic dentist in Ellicot City, MD, was giving us the lowdown on root canals. He told our group that anyone that had a root canal would have to lose the tooth. I had ten root canal teeth. I couldn't even imagine losing ten teeth, the pain of removing them and the money it would cost. So I sat on it for almost a year until I started to get my vertigo back. I then decided to start the grueling process of getting my teeth, not only pulled but all the roots would be removed and the mercury removed from my gums (mercury tattoos) and cleaned out all the way down to the bone. Most of the bone was so infected that I had to have the soft infected bone dug out. With each tooth removal, I started to feel so much better, having all of the infection removed from my body.

Dr. Sambataro has done over 1,000 studies showing that 100 percent of all of his extractions of root canal teeth were all infected. On the next page you will see a chart showing just one of my extracted teeth that had 16 different infections from just one tooth. Six of the infections were in the toxic category.

Dental DNA
5082 List Drive
Colorado Springs, CO 80919

Telephone: 719-219-2826	Fax:	719-548-8220
TIN: 84-1413291	CLIA#:	06D2019763

Lab Director: Christopher W. Shade, Ph.D, NRCC-EAC   Lab Manager: Robert C. Wheeler, BS, MS

PATIENT: DENTIST:
Lisa   Torbert   Eugene Sambataro   **Full View Test**

Sample Collected	Sample Received	Sample Tested	Test Reported
04/11/2013	04/15/2013	04/16/2013	04/16/2013

Sample Type: Tissue/Tooth #15

The following bacteria were detected in the sample that was submitted for testing:

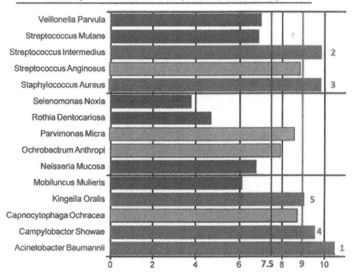

9 or greater indicates a serious risk

Greater than 7.5 but less than 9 indicates a moderate risk

Total Risk Factor, as reported on the chart above, is the sum of the Pathogen Risk Factor and Measured Risk Factor. Total Risk Factor between 7.5 and 9 is considered of moderate risk. Total Risk Factor equal to or greater than 9 is considered a serious risk.

The Pathogen Risk Factor is the innate risk of the microbe based on the biology of the organism, disease causation, and microbial antibiotic resistance. It is reported on a scale of 1-10, with 10 being most serious and 1 most benign.

The Measured Risk Factor is the value given to the sample taking into account the quantity and configuration of the pathogen DNA. It is reported on a scale of 1-10, with 10 being most serious and 1 most benign.

Interpretation of Results:
These results are from DNA PCR testing, and indicate the presence of targeted foreign DNA. The verbiage is supplied as a courtesy to health care providers to aide in an overall assessment. This information alone should not be used to diagnose or treat a health problem or disease. Consultation with a qualified health care provider is required.

I had nine teeth extracted and waited a year to have the last one out since it was near the front and I would need a bottom plate. I really thought just one root canal could not really affect my health. I was really wrong. My vertigo came back again. It started one day with a migraine and then vertigo followed and lasted six weeks. The day I had my last tooth taken out, my vertigo completely went away and has never come back.

Also, my depression went with it. I had some mild depression over the last few years that I just couldn't explain. My life was great; I am happily married, great kids and grandkids, have a business I love and a brand new house. I would wake up just feeling not quite right. It was like I had to force my happiness. I can honestly say that my happiness and health has returned. I just can't tell you how important removing bad teeth are to your complete healing. Many of you may not have root canals and may only need to have the silver/mercury removed.

As for me, I regained my health and got rid of my vertigo, migraines, depression and fibromyalgia. When I had fibromyalgia, I was crippled when I first got out of my chair and tried to walk and suffered all day with pain. My fibromyalgia disappeared after eight of my root canal teeth were removed. Just like that!

"A Bridge Over Troubled Water"

I may have lost a lot of teeth, have one bridge, an upper and lower plate, but I would not change it for the world. Most of the last seven years, I suffered silently in pain. I wonder how long those infections were brewing under my root canal teeth. I had x-rays for years and they were unable to find the hidden infections. Pockets of infections can hide under the teeth for years. The infections leak toxins into the body and start to depress the immune system. It makes sense if you think about it. You drill out the root of the tooth, killing the tooth. Then you fill it in, cut off the oxygen and create the perfect breeding ground for bacteria to grow. Then these toxins leech into the body wreaking havoc on it. No antibiotics can touch the infection under the root canals. In fact, a root canal is the only infection that cannot be cured by antibiotics. It has been suggested that toxins leaking out of the root canals can cause systemic diseases such to the heart, kidney, nervous and endocrine systems.

The following are symptoms from having mercury amalgams:

- Swollen lymph nodes
- Heart racing/palpitations
- Metallic taste in mouth
- Coated tongue
- Allergy symptoms
- Stuffy nose
- Loss of balance, vertigo
- Sore throat
- Joint pain, swelling, stiffness
- Fibromyalgia
- Chronic Fatigue
- Arthritis
- Yeast/ Candida Infection
- Depression
- Poor Memory
- Anxiety
- Headaches/Migraines
- Dry Skin
- Female and Male Hair loss
- Cold Hands and Feet

Alzheimer patients often exhibit increased concentration of heavy metals such as mercury in their blood and brain.

Multiple Sclerosis - 1987 study showed that the level of mercury in the spinal fluid of MS patients was eight times higher than normal.

Idiopathic Dilated Cardiomyopathy (IDCM) - Mercury levels in the heart tissue of individuals who died from IDCM were found to be on average 22,000 times higher than in individuals who died of other forms of heart disease.

Dental amalgam fillings are usually silver fillings that contain and release mercury, tin, copper, and silver into the body. Even though it has been proven how toxic these materials are, many dentists are still using them because they are strong and last a long time. They are also cost effective. Most silver amalgams contain 50 percent mercury. Mercury has been considered a poison since the 1500's and was introduced into dentistry in the 1800's.

Many dentists are taught and still believe that they do not transfer mercury into the body. However this is not true. The mercury can travel from the tooth to the root, imbed in the mouth or gums, to the bone, connective tissues and then to the nerves. This allows access to the central nervous system which then starts to depress the immune system and starts to destroy different areas of the body, especially the thyroid.

FDA has stated the following

"Dental amalgam contains elemental mercury. It releases low levels of mercury vapor that can be inhaled. High levels of mercury vapor exposure are associated with adverse effects in the brain and the kidneys. FDA has reviewed the best available scientific evidence to determine whether the low levels of mercury vapor associated with dental amalgam fillings are a cause for concern. Based on this evidence, FDA considers dental amalgam fillings safe for adults and children ages 6 and above. The amount of mercury measured in the bodies of people with dental amalgam fillings is well below levels associated with adverse health effects."

And then they say this:

"Dental amalgam is a restorative material that contains approximately 50% mercury in the elemental form. Mercury vapor is released from amalgam restorations, especially during mastication and brushing. A positive correlation has been shown between the levels of mercury in blood, urine, and tissues and the number of amalgam restorations."

And then this:

"Federal health officials are warning consumers not to use skin creams, beauty and antiseptic soaps, or lotions that might contain mercury. The products are marketed as skin lighteners and anti-aging treatments that remove age spots, freckles, blemishes and wrinkles, says Gary Coody, National Health Fraud Coordinator in the Food and Drug Administration's Office of Regulatory Affairs."

"Exposure to mercury can have serious health consequences," says Charles Lee, M.D., a senior medical advisor at the FDA. "It can damage the kidneys and the nervous system, and interfere with the development of the brain in unborn children and very young children." You don't have to use the product yourself to be affected, says FDA toxicologist Mike Bolger, Ph.D. "People—particularly children—can get mercury in their bodies from breathing in mercury vapors if a member of the household uses a skin cream containing mercury." Infants and small children can ingest mercury if they touch their parents who have used these products, get cream on their hands and then put their hands and fingers into their mouth, which they are prone to do, adds Bolger.

I have read a lot from the FDA site and there is so much information about mercury. It is hard to understand and can get quite complicated. I just want people to see that the FDA does see some danger with the dental use of mercury and it seems that they are in need of more studies. I personally know the danger of mercury and root canals and how it affected my health, but I also know from other clients that have been through similar experiences.

Dr. Weston Price was one of the first to recognize and document how an infection in a specific tooth can cause degeneration in the associated organ. In one study Dr. Price removed root-canal teeth from patients who had developed heart disease following a root canal procedure, and he found that the patient's heart disease improved. He later implanted the extracted root-canal teeth into healthy rabbits, and they immediately developed heart disease and died.

Why is mercury amalgams considered safe in your mouth, but there are such harsh standards to get rid of it from the EPA. My advice is to consider getting fillings that do not contain mercury…it's just a safer decision. To help keep your mouth free of unwanted bacteria, consider oil pulling which can help remove unwanted bacteria. Swish sesame oil in your mouth for 5 to 15 minutes. Remember saliva is what transports toxins to the body.

"Lure the Best" Buy Safe
Dr. Marshalls Owner of Premier Research Labs
Fish Recommendations

Even though the list below contains the mercury levels of fish and seafood, there are other considerations on how fish are caught and killed, if they are farm raised or wild caught, or what other types of feed these sea creatures ingest. The following are recommendations from Dr. Marshall from Premier Research Labs.

Most Recommended (Wild Caught)

Dover Sole

Halibut

Swai

Whitefish

Sardines

Anchovies

Cordina

Mackerel

Haddock

Red Snapper

Less Desirable
Don't Eat or Eat Less Often

Salmon

Flounder

Sea Bass

Shrimp

Tilapia

Trout

Catfish

Mahi Mahi

Cod

Herring

Shark

Tuna

Albacore

Crab

Lobster

Scallops

The following is a list of fish and seafood and their mercury contents from least to most mercury. The categories on the list were determined according to the following mercury levels in the flesh of tested fish.

- Least mercury: Less than 0.09 parts per million
- Moderate mercury: From 0.09 to 0.29 parts per million
- High mercury: From 0.3 to 0.49 parts per million
- Highest mercury: More than .5 parts per million

Least Mercury
Enjoy these fish:

Anchovies

Butterfish

Catfish

Clam

Crab (Domestic)

Crawfish/Crayfish

Croaker (Atlantic)

Flounder

Haddock (Atlantic)

Hake

Herring

Mackerel (N. Atlantic)

Mullet

Oyster

Perch (Ocean)

Plaice

Pollock

Salmon (Fresh)

Sardine

Scallop

Shad (American)

Shrimp

Sole (Pacific)

Squid (Calamari)

Tilapia

Trout (Freshwater)

Whitefish

Whiting

Moderate Mercury

Eat six servings or less per month:

Bass (Striped, Black)

Carp

Cod (Alaskan)

Croaker (White Pacific)

Halibut (Atlantic)

Halibut (Pacific)

Jacksmelt

(Silverside)

Lobster

Mahi Mahi

Monkfish

Perch (Freshwater)

Sablefish

Skate

Snapper

Tuna (Canned

chunk light)

Tuna (Skipjack)

Weakfish (Sea Trout)

High Mercury

Eat three servings or less per month:

Bluefish

Grouper

Mackerel (Spanish, Gulf)

Sea Bass (Chilean)

Tuna (Canned Albacore)

Tuna (Yellowfin)

Highest Mercury
Avoid eating:

Mackerel (King)
Marlin
Orange Roughy
Shark
Swordfish
Tilefish
Tuna (Bigeye, Ahi)

Sources for NRDC's guide: The data for this guide to mercury in fish comes from two federal agencies: the Food and Drug Administration, which tests fish for mercury, and the Environmental Protection Agency, which determines mercury levels that it considers safe for women of childbearing age.

12

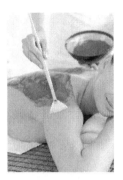

"HITS THE SPOT" DETOXING

A detox program can help the body's natural cleansing process by:

1. Resting the organs through fasting.
2. Stimulating the liver to drive toxins from the body.
3. Promoting elimination through the intestines, kidneys and skin.
4. Improving circulation of the blood.
5. Refueling the body with healthy nutrients.

The body is always trying to get rid of toxins, always detoxing through almost every organ. New research shows that almost every disease can be linked to toxicity. We live in such a toxic world, where everything around us like the air we breathe, the chemicals we clean with, the toxic chemicals used in gardening, the food we eat, what we put on our skin, and the toxins we drink.

Managing a detox system to reduce toxins during a weight program is essential for reaching your goal. Toxic excess is a major reason for weight gain, and also making it impossible to lose weight. So many things can add toxicity such as eating too much food, eating too much protein causing ammonia, also too much fat and sugar can kill off cells. As we age and the toxic load increases, it causes infection, inflammation and disease. At this point the only way we are going to heal is by using a good detox system.

The following organs will be especially critical in detoxing since they are the organs that are responsible for getting rid of toxins.

1. **Kidney:**
   Symptoms: due to the build-up of waste products in the body that may cause weakness, shortness of breath, lethargy, and confusion.
   Disease: Kidney stones, kidney infection, and kidney failure.
   Body Function and Detox: Cleans the blood of toxins and urine.
   Detox Process: Drink filtered water to keep your kidney's working well.
   Supplements: use RenaVen, Mudpack to detox the kidneys, limit or eliminate medications under a doctor's care, especially antibiotics.

2. **Liver:**
   Symptoms: liver diseases include weakness and fatigue, weight loss, nausea, vomiting, and yellow discoloration of the skin (jaundice).
   Disease: Cirrhosis occurs when normal liver cells are replaced by scar tissue.
   Body Function: The main functions of the liver are to process nutrients from food, make bile, remove toxins from the body and build protein. The liver keeps toxins from damaging the body.
   Detox Process: Limit Alcohol, Sugar and Carbs. Do Liver Mudpack Detoxes.
   Supplements: Premier Liver ND, Reishi, and HepatoVen.

3. **Lungs:**

   Symptoms: low oxygen level in blood, shortness of breath, bluish color on skin, lips and fingernails, confusion, sleepy, lose consciousness, and arrhythmias.

   Disease: Bronchitis, COPD, Asthma, Pneumonia, Influenza, Lung Cancer, Sleep Apnea, Sudden Infant Death Syndrome, Tuberculosis, etc.

   Body Function: The purpose of the lungs is to bring oxygen into the body and to remove carbon dioxide. Oxygen is a gas that provides us energy while carbon dioxide is a waste product or "exhaust" of the body.

   Detox Process: Mudpack detox the lungs front and back. Supplements: Pneumo and Chem Detox. Eliminate all associations with all types of chemical and air toxins, and quit smoking.

4. **Lymphatic System:**

   Symptoms: Constantly sick or tired.

   Disease: Lymphedema and Cancer.

   Body Function: Your lymphatic system is comprised of your lymph nodes, spleen, thymus and vessels that carry fluids to protect your body from disease. They contain white blood cells that defend against disease.

   Detox Process: Lymphatic massage and detox the lymph nodes.

   Supplements: ImmunoND.

5. **Bladder:**

   Symptoms: Infections - burning sensation, urge to urinate, cloudy or bloody urine with strong foul odor, and bladder spasms. Cancer - Pain in lower back, swelling in lower legs, growth in pelvis, pain during urination, frequent urinary tract infections, and blood clots in urine.

   Disease: Bladder Infections and Bladder Cancer.

Body Function: Urine is made in the kidneys, and travels down two tubes called ureters to the bladder. The bladder stores urine, allowing urination to be infrequent and voluntary.

Detox: The bladder works eliminating moisture accumulation in the body in the form of urine. It helps, along with the kidneys, to clean toxic buildup caused by the consumption of foods and liquids.

6. **Colon:**

   Symptoms: Diarrhea, constipation, changes in stool consistency, blood in stool, weakness, fatigue, and unexplained weight loss.

   Disease: Diverticulosis, Ulcerative Colitis, Irritable Bowel Syndrome, and Colon Cancer.

   Body Function: Absorption of water and minerals, formation and elimination of feces, contains nearly 60 varieties of friendly bacteria to aid digestion, promote vital nutrient production, to maintain pH (acid-base) balance, and to prevent proliferation of harmful bacteria.

   Detox: Eliminates toxins in the intestines. Colon Hydrotherapy and Juice Cleansing.

   Supplements: HCL, Galactin, Premier Digest, and Digestase. Mudpack to detox the intestinal area.

7. **Sweat Glands**

   According to research reported by the Centers for Disease Control and Prevention (CDC) in 2005, more than 2,000 people tested showed traces of about 60 different toxins -- including uranium and dioxins -- in their systems. Our sweat glands also get rid of toxins for us.

Detoxing is the complete process that will transform your health to the healthiest you want to be. It is an ongoing process and will depend on how much you are willing to put into it. As far as the clients I see, the sicker they are, the more they dedicate to healing. The only people who will understand this are the ones that are sick now or have been. If you have ever been really ill, especially those who have been for a long time, you know if you don't have your health, you have nothing. *"Health is not appreciated until sickness appears."*

There are many types of detoxing. The first type of detoxing is just changing your diet. If you go from a diet filled with fast foods and processed foods, including a lot of frozen meals, try adding more fruits and vegetables.

The second type of detox system is implementing a supplement program. It will nourish your body, giving you and your organs the support they need to start to transform your health. With the deficiency in our soil today, the vitamins and minerals have been depleted, so even if you try to eat well, it is just not enough. If you have abused your body with toxins like; fast food, processed food, stress, alcohol and drugs, etc., your body is so depleted for nutrients that when you add good quality supplements this will automatically throw your body into a detoxed state. Premier Research Labs supplements are organic and made with live source plants giving you healthy nutrients, vitamins and minerals. If you are using supplements currently and feel no better, know that your supplements, most likely, do not carry a strong enough nutritional value to make a difference. *"Eat the best and leave the rest."*

The third type of detoxing is the Medi Body mud pack external detox program. You will need to find a QRA practitioner to start your detox program. The number for Premier Research Labs is (800) 325-7734; they can assist in finding a practitioner in your area.

I had several operations and trauma in my 57 years of life including operations for a Hernia, Syringomyelia, Tonsils, tubes in my ears, (3) D & C, Urethra dilation and an Appendectomy. I also broke my arm, was in two car accidents, tore cartilage in my knee, had a baby, and 25 years of being a pin cushion from allergy shots. I had to detox from all of my operations and a lifetime of abuse to my body. More than half of my healing definitely came from the mud pack detox system. Although there were days that I felt sick from the detox, I would do it all over again in a minute. To get up each day and feel good is such a blessing. I realize that most of you will not have as many diseases, and aliments as I had, so your healing will be much faster and easier. But there will be those who will be able to relate to the pain, suffering and frustration they have had where no doctor could fix them. I have cured from all of my diseases and aliments. I feel I am obligated to pass on what I have learned as people can relate and empathize with my personal experiences. There were times when I thought, "How can I endure through one more disease?" "Why am I getting one disease after another?" Who is this sick? I have always been a very strong person both mentally and physically, but there were times when I wondered if I could get through all of this. I now realize that it was a blessing. I was able to heal through all of this naturally and my gift is that I can write about it and share this with you. "*Stay strong to Live Long*"

I wanted to share a couple of detox sessions from one of my 80 year old clients. She had a kidney removed when she was a teenager. I first detoxed the scar area where she had the kidney removed. She had very strong detox symptoms for most of that day, where she was totally exhausted and slept most of the day. The next day I detoxed her other kidney, which I thought would produce worse detox symptoms since her one kidney had to work so hard her entire life. I was surprised to find that she had no detox symptoms at all from the kidney still in her body. In fact she felt great. This goes to show you that when an organ is removed from the body it is so important to detox that area. When an area of the body is cut open toxins will start to accumulate in the disturbed area of the body. For my client, it had been 60 years of accumulated toxins that were removed and she felt better than she had in years.

Are you ready to start your detox program?

Premier Medi-Body Pack is applied externally, draws out deeply embedded toxins from Operation sites, Injury sites, Interference sites, Organs, Sinus areas and more. It quickly eliminates the build-up of these hidden toxins, helps increase circulation, boosts the immune system, eases muscle tension, and rejuvenates cells.

This is one of the most important parts to healing. If you have had surgeries, injection sites, piercings, tattoos, burns, sprains, falls, whiplash, radiation, metal objects surgically added, etc., this system will safely detox those areas of trauma. Quantum-state "mud" packs contain unheated volcanic clay, peat magma and Indian Shilajit. It promotes cleansing and bio-energetic flow and initiates the "thermal effect," a deep intrinsic cleansing effect.

What are Interference sites?

A key factor overlooked in literally every disease or sickness is hidden deep-seated toxicity deep within the body causing interference sites, which prevents normal nerve and energy flow (chi). These embedded toxins can mean years of delayed healing - or none at all. The interference fields include any area where the skin has been cut or pierced. This includes C-sections, episiotomies, any operation, vaccination sites, allergy shot sites, ear or body piercings, tattoos, and dental surgeries. Other areas to detox may include injuries from a fall or accident, such as a broken bone, whiplash from a car accident, a burn, sprain, radiation, and surgically-added metal objects. These interference sites prevent normal nerve and energy flow, making it a toxic dump area where toxins build up around the site. It seems logical that when we injure an area, even as a child, that area becomes weaker over time if we do not remove the toxins.

Detoxing is one of the most effective parts to healing. One way to detox is to find a QRA practitioner that can detox you using the Medi Body Pack System, a deep healing mud applied externally to different parts of the body. When detoxing with a QRA practitioner, they will test the areas of trauma and find out where they are reflecting to. A reflect point, or a chakra, is a center of vital energy that aligns with the spine. You will then be given a detoxifying drink to help keep your body strong during the detox. The detox mud will then be applied to two sites on the body; the injury and the reflecting point. An "Earthwrappe" infrared heating pad will then be applied on top of one or both of the sites to speed up the detoxifying process. You will be covered up so that you can remain warm and comfortable during your detox. Most of my clients sleep the entire hour of the detox.

Another way to detox your body is by doing castor oil packs. I use Premier's Caster Oil and Organic Cotton along with my Earthwrappe. The Earthwrappe is important because it's job is to pull toxins out of the body via the infrared system. The great part about the castor oil packs is that you can do them in the privacy of your own home. Here are the instructions for use:

1. Place your organic cotton in a glass bowl and pour castor oil over it.
2. Wear old clothes since the oil will stain your clothes
3. Place the castor oil cotton on the desired spot. Place a clean piece of cotton next to the oiled one
4. Place a non- toxic clear plastic over it.
5. Place your Earthwrappe, hot water bottle or heating pad next to the plastic. Keep it on for 60 minutes.
6. When finished, throw the cotton away. The cotton now contains the toxins from the affected area.
7. After the detox, I like to use Premier's Medi Body Bath. I go outside, weather permitting, and submerge my feet into the water to help speed up the detox process. I soak for 10 to 15 minutes.

This process is recommended to use daily, especially if you are really toxic.

"No Pain...No Gain"

When you are coming in for a detox session and starting on a supplement program you most likely will have detox symptoms. I had a few people discontinue early in their healing because they were afraid of the detox symptoms also because they felt worse. This is crucial to understand that the toxins are being released from your body. These symptoms usually last a few hours. However, this is proof that the toxins are starting to come out of your organs and into the bloodstream.

Research has shown us that when you do lose weight, toxins are released from stored fat and enter into your bloodstream. Women have a higher percentage of body fat, so their bodies may hold more toxins in the fat. When we lose weight, we expose our organs now to toxicity, since our fat was protecting our organs from these toxins.

You may experience detox symptoms such as:

1. Sick to your stomach
2. Headache
3. Extremely tired (hours to days)
4. Pain in kidneys
5. Diarrhea
6. Swelling and retaining water

If you give up caffeine you can also experience detox symptoms, since you are ridding your body of toxins/drugs. The detox and/or supplement program may start to detox your body the same way. The more toxic, the more detoxing your body will need.

Here is a list of things that make the body more toxic:

1. Taking medications
2. Surgeries
3. Eating junk foods (sugar, cakes, cookies)
4. Poor digestion
5. Poor dental health
6. Hormonal imbalance

So let's recap…if you feel sick during your mud detox, you are removing toxins and that is a good thing (it will pass). Detox symptoms normally last a few hours. Once I detoxed a cancer patient and she had a full day of detox symptoms. So, of course, it will depend on how sick you are. If you detox too quickly then we can always slow things down. If you have a terminal disease, then we would need to stay with the program and make your detox program an aggressive one. Remember it took years of toxicity to get you here, so you need to be patient as it will take some time to bring you back. Try to enjoy the journey, knowing a healthy you is in your future. Detoxification is a central component in long-term effective weight management.

13

"I'M THINKING DIFFERENT, I'M THINKING QRA"

A re you tired of being sick? Tired of being told it is all in your head? Tired of being offered antidepressants? Did you know prescription drugs only treat the symptoms? Do you catch colds often? Have flu and allergy symptoms? Just don't feel good?

Do you suffer from: Low Energy, Trouble Sleeping, Depression, Hormonal imbalance, Ear infections, Sore throats, Sinus trouble, Adrenal Fatigue, Crones, Rashes, Nail Fungus, Fibromyalgia, Indigestion, Heartburn, Gas & Bloating?

What if your body could talk to you and tell you what was wrong and what you needed to be healthy? Did you know that it can through Quantum Reflex Analysis (QRA), a unique, highly effective testing of the bio-energetic status of the body's key organs and glands? It uses a university proven muscle testing technique of <u>medically accepted</u> reflex points. QRA can quickly pinpoint problem areas to determine the precise nutrients and exact amounts needed to rapidly restore your energy and dramatically improve your health. QRA has the ability to identify and eliminate the "<u>root of the problem</u>." Practitioners use specific testing techniques to identify hidden infections that may be causing ill health from interference sites from traumas, surgeries, improper eating habits, stress, etc. In just one session, your practitioner can determine what key organs are deficient and provide you with an overall assessment and program to get you started on a new state of health.

You will learn how your individual body communicates its needs through the language of QRA. Our bodies have a magnificent internal intelligence that can rejuvenate the body and return the endurance, vitality, peak mental and physical performance and health that we all enjoyed in our younger years. Your body can talk to you through an amazing bio-communication technique called QRA. It includes specific testing techniques to find hidden infections, hormone imbalance, thyroid imbalance, digestive problems, skin rashes, and heart trouble, just to name a few. QRA can also find deficiencies in vitamins such as B, D and Calcium.

Your QRA Practitioner will test acupuncture meridians on the surface of your body. You will need to have strength in your hands or call your practitioner ahead of time so that they may provide a surrogate to help assist during the test. You will be asked to create an "O-ring" with your fingers and place a finger of your other hand directly onto the acupuncture meridian point(s). This technique is painless, simple and easy to perform. Once the practitioner has determined which organs/glands need help, they will test nutrients or formulas to find the exact match your body needs. Your body will actually pick the supplements and the amounts needed to nourish unhealthy organs and glands back to health. I have treated over 200 chronically ill, fatigued, and diseased patients, teaching everyone the secrets of regeneration and healing though organic supplementation, external detoxing and proper nutrition.

The Truth about Toxins

QRA treatments are a natural way of boosting up the immune system so it can safely remove a lifetime of toxins from our bodies. These toxins can come from eating nutrient deficient foods such as: junk foods, fast foods, prepackaged foods, meats and dairy products containing antibiotics, pesticides and growth hormones. It may also come from bad lifestyle choices such as smoking, alcohol consumption, and/or consuming illegal and prescription medications. Surgical procedures can also leave hidden scars and toxins that impede optimal functioning. Environmental toxins such as heavy metals, air, water, land and chemical pollution and vector borne illnesses such as Lyme disease or Babesia, are just few of the many other environmental dangers that we are potentially exposed to on a regular basis.

"It's Electric"

Let's face it, most of us work on computers, carry smart phones, use microwaves and other devices daily that contain electromagnet fields (EMF), which is an intrusion to our bodies. The health effects from EMF products include decreased immune function, increased blood pressure, impaired nervous system function, cancers and brain damage. There have been many new cases of breast cancers in teenagers who carry their cell phones in their bras. It is time to protect yourself.

You can purchase several devices for your protection from the effects of EMF. Premier offers a Q-Disc which is an ultra-thin polarity disc for all cell-phones, including iPhones. You install this device on the back of your phone for your daily protection. I have a Q-Disc on my phone and keep it near me when I work on my computer for extra protection. Did you know that a 30 second cell phone call can weaken every cell in your body? The Q-Disk protects you from the EMFs and also converts the harmful field into a beneficial field.

Also, I recommend the Pyra Fire Pyramid for home, business and car use. This pyramid creates a strong coherent field which transforms the depolarizing energy into a healing, beneficial energy that strengthens and protects us from all EMFs. I bring one in the car, and on airplanes, and especially when I stay in a hotel where the room is buzzing with all types of interference. You are not only protecting yourself from the EFA effects, you are changing the energy into a more peaceful environment. When people come into my center they remark about how good it feels. This is amazing that even people that do not understand energy can feel the effects of it. This is an important purchase that you need to make to continue your health journey.

Did you know that everything has energy? Not just humans, but plants, wood, glass, stones, etc. Quantum physics shows us that everything has a different amount of energy, and this energy can be either good or bad. When I test glass it has a very strong energy, but when I test a plastic bag it has a very bad energy. The QRA test can not only test the body, it can test anything in the world. The loss of energy or strength of energy in your body from the Q-ring test will show what type of energy the item has.

Quantum physics is the study of the behavior of matter and energy at the molecular, atomic, nuclear, and even smaller microscopic levels. The birth of quantum physics is attributed to Max Planck's 1900 paper on blackbody radiation. Development of the field was done by Max Planck, Albert Einstein and many other scientists. Energy is real!

14

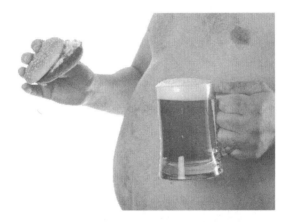

"THINK OUTSIDE THE BUN" TOXICITY IN FAT

How do you Roll? Are you a Muffin Top? Have a Buddha Belly?
Beer Belly? Jelly Belly?

I think we can all agree that "muffin tops," the fat hanging over the waist, and beer bellies aren't very attractive and they are everywhere. We really don't want to look like that. Don't you get sick of all the things you have tried to get rid of belly fat? How about the advertisements, infomercials, magazine ads and television shows telling you to try this one product to get rid of belly fat. You buy one, go to the gym and do 100 crunches and nothing works. That is because it is much more complicated than a magic potion that someone is selling. If it looks too good to be true, guess what? It probably is! We know that excess belly fat has been linked to diabetes, cardiovascular disease, and some cancers. It's dangerous and we can't seem to do anything about it.

In 2008, I weighed a whopping 191 pounds, an all-time high. When I think about it I never even got to enjoy eating yummy fattening foods. My diet was basically the same and I still gained 50 pounds within a year, without overeating. Now, after detoxing and taking supplements from Premier Research Labs, I have healed and lost 40 of the 50 pounds. When I lost the weight, I noticed that even though I weighed the same as I did ten years ago, I now have a pouch. So the million dollar question is why do so many people have belly fat? Many think it is age. I can tell you, it is not! I will attempt to give you the easiest breakdown of the science behind belly fat....Toxins!

"If a Bug Won't Bite it, Why Should You"

Try a little experiment. Set out a plate of margarine and another with real butter. See where the bugs go. I noticed online several people tried this experiment. The ants were all over the butter and there were none on the margarine. Since it is wintertime in Delaware, I was not able to get any results from the experiment, since no critters were out at this time.

Chemicals, Pesticides, Food Additives are Everywhere

The U.S. Environmental Protection Agency (EPA) has estimated that approximately 750,000 chemicals are now in use in homes, industry, and agriculture. This does not include pesticides, pharmaceuticals, and food additives, or the estimated 1,500 different ingredients used

in pesticides (Geyer et al. 1986). Dioxins are environmental pollutants. They belong to the so-called "dirty dozen" - a group of dangerous chemicals known as persistent organic pollutants (POPs).

Old news: 100 percent of toxins in everyone's body fat

First of all, there was a study completed in 1972 by the EPA which was monitoring human exposure to toxic environmental chemicals called the National Human Adipose Tissue Survey. This study evaluates the levels of various toxins in the fat tissue that was collected from 100 cadavers and elective surgeries. Five of the most toxic chemicals were found in **100% of all fat samples**, dioxin being one. So in 1972 we knew that toxins were in the fat of every person tested. In 1982 and again in 1987 the EPA again analyzed human fat samples from cadavers, looking for the types of toxins that live in human fat tissue. Four industrial solvents and one dioxin were found in 100 percent of the fat samples. Nine more chemicals, including three more dioxins were found in more than 90 percent of the fat samples.

Dioxins and related chemical compounds are toxic industrial pollutants which are ubiquitous and persistent in the environment, and which accumulate in the fat tissue of animals and humans. Foods of animal origin are the primary source of human exposure to dioxins. In June 2000, the EPA completed a ten-year effort to reassess the science base associated with dioxins and closely related compounds and their associated risks to human health. The draft dioxin reassessment concludes that dioxins are a human carcinogen and that the lifetime cancer risk associated with the average person's body burden of dioxin is between 1 in 100 and 1 in 1000. This estimate of risk is ten times higher than the EPA's previous estimate and represents a very significant public health concern. Animals are thought to accumulate background levels of dioxin primarily through ingestion of contaminated vegetation grown in contaminated soil. Human daily intake of dioxin and dioxin-like compounds occurs in over 90% of the foods of animal origin.

Measured dioxins in pooled food samples that were collected in 1995 at supermarkets across the U.S., Toxic Equivalents (TEQ) are:

Fresh water fish (farm raised) (1.43 TEQ1),
Butter (1.07 TEQ)
Hotdog/bologna (0.54 TEQ)
Ocean fish (0.47 TEQ)
Cheese (0.40 TEQ)
Beef (0.38 TEQ)
Eggs (0.34 TEQ)

WHY CAN'T I LOSE WEIGHT? TOXINS

Ice cream (0.33 TEQ)
Chicken (0.32 TEQ)
Pork (0.32 TEQ)
Milk (0.12 TEQ)
Vegetables, fruits, grains and legumes (0.07 TEQ)

A person's intake of dioxins through the diet therefore, depends on the relative intake of foods with high or low levels of contamination and the quantity consumed. For example, Patandin et al. (1999) investigated the dietary intake of a group of preschool children in The Netherlands and found that dairy products contributed about 50% of their intake of dioxins and related compounds, while meat/meat products and processed foods contributed about 20% - 25%, respectively.

Conclusion: We all have toxins in our fat so what does this mean?

Researchers have confirmed the presence of these different toxins inside our fatty tissue. So as we age we acquire more and more toxins until we get to the point that we will not be able to lose any weight at all, no matter what we do. I tried everything; 600 calories, 1200 calories, 1400 calories, working out and nothing worked. The toxins are stored in our fat to protect the toxins from entering our liver, heart, lungs and nervous system. The fat especially targets the belly area, and for most of us, who never had belly fat, now do. Our bodies are very intelligent. The toxins continue to spread and fill up the fat cells trying desperately to keep the toxins away from our organs. This will cause easy weight gain as your fat holds on tightly to the toxic fat it has stored.

When a person already has too many toxins, the body has nowhere else to put them so it makes new fat cells and stores the new toxins along with the fat. The new formed fat cells are also damaged by toxins and they change and slow down our metabolic process and are not able to make leptin normally. The body is so intelligent it will do everything possible to keep the toxins/poison away from the organs. This is why it is so hard to lose weight.

Toxins are fat soluble, which means they accumulate in white adipose tissue. Since they are fat soluble, the liver cells need to turn them into water soluble in order to excrete them from the body. This process makes the liver work overtime so it is important to support the liver with supplements such as Liver ND or Reishi from Premier.

Toxins make us feel tired, irritable and just plain lousy. When we change our diet and start to detox we feel even worse, tired, more irritable and add in flu like symptoms. This can be a viscous cycle because when you stop your diet and start eating toxic foods again, the toxins are pulled out of the blood and put back into the fat along with more fat and toxins. At first you might feel better, but then you go back to feeling lousy because you just keep putting more and more toxic fat and poisons into your body.

As we all know our environment is flooded with chemicals from the air, water and our food. There is no escape from these toxins. As we age, our bodies have more trouble fighting off these toxins. Try making the following changes:

- Eat organic foods
- Avoid pesticides, herbicides, hormones and antibiotics.
- Drink filtered water (reverse osmosis or carbon filter).
- HEPA/ULPA filters and ionizers can be helpful in reducing
- dust, molds, volatile organic compounds, and other sources of indoor air pollution.
- Clean and monitor heating systems for release of carbon monoxide.
- Have houseplants that help filter the air.
- Keep your window cracked at night to get fresh air.
- Air out your dry cleaning before wearing it.
- Avoid excess exposure to environmental petrochemicals (garden chemicals, dry cleaning, car exhaust, second-hand smoke).
- Avoid heavy metals that cause the most ill health such as: lead, mercury, cadmium, arsenic, nickel, and aluminum.
- Avoid chemical toxins including volatile organic compounds (VOCs), solvents (cleaning materials, formaldehyde, toluene, benzene).

🐦 Avoid medications, pesticides, herbicides, and food additives.

🐦 Infections (hepatitis C virus) and mold toxins.

🐦 Avoid sugar, high-fructose corn syrup, trans fatty acids, alcohol.

🐦 Avoid caffeine, tobacco and aspartame.

🐦 Do not use genetically modified organisms (GMOs) or non BPA free plastics.

🐦 Avoid hormones and antibiotics found in our food supply.

🐦 Avoid heavy metal exposure mercury from fish and dental amalgams (silver fillings).

🐦 Avoid Vaccines and Flu Shots (loaded with chemicals).

🐦 Avoid aluminum in deodorants, antacids, and baking powder.

🐦 Avoid canned goods.

"Seven Days without Exercise Makes one Weak"

It is important to convince the body to burn fat. We need to exercise using weights to keep our muscles strong. It does not mean we need to lift incredibly heavy weights; just lift. Our fat metabolism is the body's detox fuel and it is critical that we flush these fat cells in order to remove toxins. You will need to burn fat to burn toxins. Again always consult a physician to make sure you are ready. Many will want to start out with walking and yoga and work up to it.

Cortisol and Belly Fat

Did you know that cortisol stores fat in our belly? Fat cells in the abdomen have more cortisol activating enzymes than fat in other parts of the body. There are cortisol receptors in the blood flow in abdominal fat.

Why is Fiber the Answer?

Extra body weight is linked to a survival strategy that may actually be protecting your body from higher levels of digestive damage than you would otherwise experience if you were not craving excess food. Protect your digestive system, your immune system, by adding lots of healthy fiber. Fiber acts like a sponge for toxins and gobbles them up like a giant pacman. Try 40 – 60 grams of fiber per day, using supplementation with Premiers; Galactin and Premier

Greens to help detox the intestinal area. Make a great shake and add these two ingredients.

Cortisol regulates energy by selecting a (carbohydrate, fat or protein) that is needed by the body to meet its needs at the time. An effect of the stress response is to break down fat cells to move triglycerides into the bloodstream for more energy delivering it to a working muscle. Under stressful conditions, cortisol can provide the body with protein for energy production, but **when we stay stressed out it can move fat from storage and relocate it to fat cell deposits deep in the abdomen.** It's normal for your cortisol levels to go up and down throughout the day, but when you are chronically stressed your cortisol level goes up — and stays there.

Basically, to sum it up quickly, every time you have a stress reaction (feel stressed, adrenaline rush, panic attack, feeling anxious, fight or flight response, etc.) your body secretes cortisol (hormone). I know personally, that when I get these anxious stressed feelings, my body is secreting too much cortisol and this can have a potentially devastating effect on my body. So basically, too much cortisol equals feeling like crap both mentally and physically and your body will hold on to belly fat. Double whammy!

The consequences of excess cortisol causes
Abdominal obesity
high blood sugar (adrenal diabetes)
muscle wasting
bone loss
immune shutdown
thin wrinkled skin
fluid retention
hypertension

Excessive cortisol frequently causes increased: Fatigue/decreased energy, irritability, impaired memory, depressed mood, decreased libido, hormone imbalance, insomnia, anxiety, impaired concentration, fears and phobias.

Chronically high cortisol may contribute to many diseases, including cancer, ulcers, heart attacks, diabetes, infections, alcoholism, strokes, skin diseases, psychosis, multiple sclerosis, myasthenia gravis, and possibly Parkinson's and Alzheimer's disease. High Cortisol may contribute to obesity not only because of the metabolic disruptions (including insulin resistance) that it promotes, but also because it induces "stress over-eating," especially in women. It weakens your immune system and makes you more susceptible to getting sick.

Ways to Reduce High Cortisol:

1. Use cortisol reducing supplement: Premiers Melatonin and Tranquinol.
2. Eat at regular intervals throughout the day. Avoid skipping meals, as this will create a cortisol release.
3. Excessive carbohydrate intake creates cortisol release in response to constantly elevated insulin levels. Eat complex carbohydrates instead.
4. Utilize stress reduction techniques at peak cortisol times: meditation, self-hypnosis, or deep breathing exercises.
5. Get to bed on time at 10:00 pm if possible. Get at least seven to eight hours of sleep nightly.
6. Avoid stimulants: Stay away from energy drinks that contain ephedra-like compounds and caffeine. Stimulants can also disrupt your sleeping patterns. If you must drink coffee or sodas be sure that you do not drink any after 12 noon. Coffee needs to be organic.
7. Keep your workouts to an hour or less. Cortisol rises after an hour and puts more stress on the body.
8. Eat foods that reduce cortisol; Salmon, halibut, walnuts, drink black tea, eat dark chocolate and citrus such as bell peppers, fruits, and leafy green vegetables.

"Hormones and Body Fat "Chemical Calories"

Paula F Baillie-Hamilton MB BS DPhil (Occupational and Environmental Health Research Group at Stirling University, Stirling, Scotland), an expert on metabolism and the impact of toxins upon the human system, has proposed that toxins in our environment may lie at the cause of weight gain.

Dr. Baillie-Hamilton has, through years of research, identified certain toxic chemicals, which can cause a person to gain weight. She calls these substances 'Chemical Calories' because they act within our bodies as hormones, and have a damaging effect on the sympathetic nervous system (SNS), the hormonal regulatory system for weight control. Dr. Baillie-Hamilton defines a 'Chemical Calorie' as an estimated value of the degree of damage caused by a chemical to our natural weight loss systems.

When you have stress, your body releases certain "fight-or-flight" stress hormones that are produced in the adrenal glands: cortisol, norepinephrine and epinephrine. When you first get stressed, these hormones kick into gear. Norepinephrine tells your body to stop producing insulin so that you can have plenty of fast-acting blood glucose ready. Epinephrine will relax the muscles in your stomach and intestines and decrease blood flow to these organs. Once the stressor has passed, cortisol tells the body to stop producing these hormones and to go back to digesting regularly. When your stress and cortisol levels are high, the body actually resists weight loss. Your body thinks times are hard and you might starve, so it hoards the fat you eat or have present on your body. Cortisol tends to take fat from healthier areas, like your butt and hips, and move it to your abdomen which has more cortisol receptors. In the process, it turns once–healthy peripheral fat into unhealthy visceral fat (the fat in your abdomen that surrounds your organs) that increases inflammation and insulin resistance in the body. This belly fat then leads to more cortisol because it has higher concentrations of an enzyme that converts inactive cortisone to active cortisol. The more belly fat you have, the more active cortisol will be converted by these enzymes, yet another vicious cycle created by visceral fat.

15

"SUGAR & SPICE, NOTHING NICE" INFLAMMATION & INFECTIONS

One of the first signs of toxic fat in your body is gaining weight without an increase in food or a reduction of exercise. Toxic body fat causes chronic inflammation in the body.

Chronic inflammation is the body's response to toxins:

Environmental toxins (air, water, food, mercury in teeth)

Emotional toxicity (excessive worrying and stress)

Physical stress (workaholic, excessive exercise)

Food toxicity (sugar, carbohydrates, fat, junk food, non-organic foods)

The first signs of a metabolic change in the body are that many people get diabetes and high cholesterol. This is only the beginning of the deterioration of our health. The toxins that were safely contained in your fat are now leeching into your body and attacking your organs and immune system. Many men and especially women start to gain weight between the ages of 45 and 55. The toxins spread into the fat and we begin to gain the weight as a protective barrier to prevent the spread of toxins into the organs. When we continue to load our body with endless amounts of toxins from unhealthy foods, the fat starts to escape and causes the development of disease from cancer to fibromyalgia. Chronic disease takes years of toxic abuse to form. The biggest form of inflammation is chronic pain. I will say that chronic pain is one of the hardest things to conquer, but as you remove the hidden infections in your body, you will heal. Most of us already have inflammation and do not know it.

Visible signs of inflammation and Autoimmune Disease include:

Bacterial infections	Urinary tract infections
Fungal infections	Acid reflux
Viral infections	Cancer
Arthritis	Skin conditions psoriasis and acne
Bronchitis	Thyroid conditions
Chronic pain	Lupus
Diabetes	Allergies
High blood pressure	Fibromyalgia
Osteoporosis	Crohn's
Candidiasis	ADHD

When I look at the list above, I notice that I had almost everything on this list. I was diagnosed with fibromyalgia and had it for two years and it was the hardest thing on the list to heal from. However, with my organic diet and removal of all my infected root canal teeth cured my fibromyalgia completely.

Look at how Diabetes Has Grown

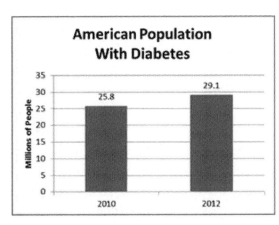

People w/ Diabetes in 1893 - 3 in 100,000
People w/ Diabetes in 2012 - 8,000 in 100,000
People in US with Diabetes in 2012 29.1%
15.5 Million Men w/diabetes in 2012
13.4 Million Women w/ diabetes in 2012

Diabetes among race 2010 – 2012, age 20 and older

Non-Hispanic Whites 7.6%

Asians 9%

Hispanics 12.9%

Non-Hispanic Blacks 13.2%

American Indians and Alaska Natives 15.9%

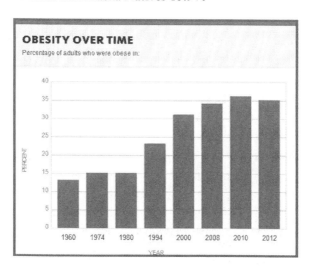

"Eat Fresh" 10 Foods That Reduce Inflammation and Pain Naturally

There are so many people that live everyday with chronic pain. I was living the life of a crippled person. When I stood up I limped. The pain was excruciating. My fibromyalgia was with me as soon as I woke up and until I went to bed. I did a juice feast for 21 days, drinking a gallon of fresh made juice a day and my fibromyalgia went away completely. However, as soon as I went back to eating regular food, the pain came back. The problem being, I still had my toxic teeth. This showed how strong raw, cold compressed juice was; like a shot of liquid vitamins, can be to treat pain and disease. If you have toxic teeth you are still going to need to have your root canal teeth removed or mercury removed for your teeth to get rid of pain and be able to heal completely.

Supplements to Help Treat Inflammation

1. **Alfalfa -** Rich in vitamins, protein and minerals. Alfalfa is naturally anti-arthritic, due to its high Chlorophyll content.
2. **Chamomile** - Natural relaxant, anti-spasmodic and an anti- inflammatory. Drink as an herbal tea.
3. **Fenugreek** - Anti-inflammatory and has phyto-steroid properties to help rebuild tissues, commonly used to season curry. Eat the plant's leaves, sprouts and seeds.
4. **Flax -** Omega 3 fatty acids anti-inflammatory properties. Make sure you grind up the seeds to release the active ingredients.
5. **Ginger** - Stimulates blood flow for improved circulation, anti- inflammatory. Do not consume ginger if you are on blood thinners.
6. **Licorice Root -** Anti-inflammatory and is rich in phyto-steroids. Limit your consumption.
7. **Salmon —** Contains Omega three fatty acids and anti-inflammatory properties to treat arthritis.
8. **Rosemary -** Naturally eases nerve and muscle tension and pain. Contains salicin, which is a natural form glycoside which aspirin is made from.
9. **Sage -** Anti-inflammatory which helps improve achy muscles and inflammation.
10. **Shitake mushroom -** Used to treat immune deficiency, anti-viral helps treat chronic joint pain and arthritis.

16

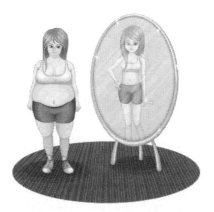

"MIRROR, MIRROR" HYPNOTHERAPY

irror, mirror on the wall, who's the fattest of them all? I was actually pretty thin in my twenties but my mind set at the time was so distorted I thought I was fat. I also had men telling me I was too fat! I was never happy with myself. I can also remember my dad was always on a diet, talking out loud about his weight. The things we subconsciously pick up and don't even realize it until we are older. My son picked up the same things from me...toxic body language.

Counseling is a wonderful way to clear out the demons that haunted us in childhood and intrude into our current life. Of course, the name calling sticks out clearly. I learned early on that boys did not like fat. This left emotional scars so deep, that I would spend my entire life doing everything in my power to be thin. That meant drugs or anything I could get my hands on to force weight loss. I did everything possible to be thin; amphetamines, ephedra and caffeine supplements and diuretics. However, when I was in my forties, I noticed things that worked in the past, no longer were working. I had developed a tolerance to losing weight, just like an addict who needs more and more to keep their fix. The worst feeling in my life was when I turned 50 and no matter how little I ate, or how much I exercised, I could not lose weight. When you lose your control or power to achieve a goal as strong as weight loss, you start to lose your mind, especially when this is what defines you. I could not go back to being overweight. I dreamt of the "good ole days," when I was thin and remembered how free I felt, how happy and normal.

Now there's my husband who has great self-esteem and a good sense of humor. He walks around rubbing his belly saying "A body like this doesn't just happen, you have to work at it." He does not care in the least that he has a belly. I think women are much more obsessed with their weight and body image than men are. Women are definitely more critical and their perceptions about their bodies are not always healthy.

When I was 45, I went back to college and decided while I worked full time at my holistic health center, that I would enroll in college full time too… just like a good little addict. In four years, I had my Masters in Community Counseling. I learned about myself and all the nasty little secrets that I forced down deep into my body. I still used my exercise addictions, worka-holic addiction and my addiction to stress, or norepinephrine addiction, to keep me thin. However, this degree saved and changed my life forever. I also went back for additional counseling; vomiting all the emotional toxins out of my body. You see, these are toxins too. They do as much harm as the foods we eat.

Years later I discovered the world of hypnotherapy. So, not like I wasn't doing enough already, I became fascinated with the results. I immediately made an appointment, for hypnotherapy, for weight loss and saw how strong it was and how it would immediately reduce my cravings for sweets. It also helped my self-esteem, it was like a speeded up counseling session. I enrolled in a hyp-notherapy course and bam, next thing you know I'm a hypnotherapist. I have helped so many people with hypnosis for weight loss, cravings for foods, to stop smoking, anxiety and most of all an increase in self-esteem.

Hypnosis for Weight Loss

Hypnosis is a powerful, proven program which taps into the power of the sub-conscious mind. You can re-program your sub-conscious to help you change your eating patterns, give you motivation to exercise, eat healthier, drink more water, and enjoy doing it. Hypnosis is the perfect tool for re-educating your sub-conscious mind, the part that creates cravings and impulses.

If you are struggling with weight loss, hypnosis can provide the extra motivation and enable you to escape the many food traps that get in the way of weight loss. Permanent weight loss occurs with a change in lifestyle, not through unnatural diets that are impossible to maintain. Hypnosis can help you make those changes, quickly and more easily than you ever imagined possible. Anyone who has been on a diet knows the powerful motivation you feel when you first start out. Then, as time goes on, the rate of weight loss slows down; you lose weight more slowly, and may even gain a bit. And suddenly, it isn't quite as easy to stay motivated any more. Hypnosis helps maintain the motivation for weight loss, keeps you feeling confident that you can achieve your perfect weight goal.

Can anyone benefit from using hypnosis?

There is good news! Using modem hypnosis techniques anyone who can follow instructions can experience the benefits of hypnosis.

Hypnosis is a naturally occurring state of mind. You have already experienced it many times. Hypnosis happens spontaneously when we find ourselves daydreaming. Another common example is what is called highway hypnosis. This occurs when you find that you have been driving for a while and you miss your turn off. You had been so focused on some other idea that you forgot to turn. Hypnosis simply helps you to use these natural human abilities to make the kind of changes you want to make, like breaking habits or improving how you feel about yourself.

Be assured, hypnosis is safe. The American Medical Association sanctioned the use of hypnosis in 1958. Since then, it has been used by millions of people worldwide. Hypnotherapists commonly receive referrals from medical and psychological professionals, in order to help their clients and patients. Since hypnosis is a consensual process (no one can be hypnotized against their will), the client is always in control and can emerge from the process at any time.

What most people know about hypnosis probably is "stage hypnosis" where the power of hypnosis is used to make people do foolish things that make the audience laugh. This takes special training for the hypnotherapist where they are able to pick those that will be hypnotized very deeply, making for a better show. However, hypnotherapy is no joke, when the power of hypnosis is unleashed, it can be used to help people heal and change their lives positively in a private session. Just think about all that power being used *to help* people. That's exactly why "modern hypnosis is called the new vogue."

During a session with a certified hypnotherapist, the subconscious mind takes over. Using the power of hypnosis, the hypnotherapist is able to deal with the subconscious mind without the interference of the "critical factor" the part of your mind that keeps reminding you that "you'll never be a success" or "you'll never lose weight." Without being criticized, the subconscious mind, which is like a library of everything that ever happened to you in your entire life, is able to deal with painful situations that are causing you problems today. Those problems may manifest as smoking, being overweight, phobias, and lack of confidence, drinking alcohol or any other harmful behaviors. If you have ever over-reacted to a situation in your life, it is because of that old pain that you are trying to hold down. Everyone has some kind of fear; we are all human, well maybe most of us. Let hypnotherapy assist you in becoming the successful, happy person that you were originally meant to be!

You Can Lose Weight with Hypnosis

The major problem with diets is that they are a major change of eating habit patterns. The main goal is to achieve the weight goal. After the diet, most of us just want to return to what we call normal eating. So the celebration begins; we reward ourselves with **cookies, pasta, pizza, chocolate,** etc. At this point there often begins an upward weight trend which can recover all of the lost weight and even pick up a few extra pounds. (Example: Atkins diet, eating no carbs to eating every carb in sight)

Why do we overeat?

Overeating usually fills a need. Some people overeat to compensate for an unpleasant experience. Others eat excessively to reward themselves or simply for self-entertainment. Some want to be noticed, feel a lack of love, to offset fear, overcome frustration, boredom, stress or even to avoid sex.

Maybe it's not the Diet but Our Attitudes and Thoughts

Changing thoughts and attitudes of the mind can lead to major changes in our life. Hypnosis will deal with such behaviors as establishing times, places and patterns for future eating, elimination of harmful habits and positive reinforcement for changing what our particular overeating problems are. During hypnosis, your food interests and tastes will be modified to increase the desire for healthy foods, for extra energy to start an exercise program, or to help eliminate craving foods such as carbs, chocolate, salted snacks and sugary treats. With hypnosis, clients desire and consume a much lesser amount of food without giving up their favorite foods and drink. Hypnosis can help clients feel more full, more satisfied after eating a small amount of a desired food, enjoying the quality, not the quantity.

"Psychological Cravings" Comfort Foods

Many of us are emotional eaters, so let's find out why. One of the biggest soothers is chocolate. Most chocolate (milk chocolate) is very unhealthy with a lot of sugar, caffeine and unhealthy oils. On the other hand, dark chocolate is low on the glycemic index and can help stabilize blood sugar levels. Chocolate can give us quick energy, lift our moods, increase serotonin in your brain, and reduce anxiety. Sugar contains a feel good ingredient called anandamide, which is also produced naturally in the brain and stimulates the same neurotransmitters that THC (the principal active chemical in marijuana) does.

Many people eat their way to relaxation and calmness by consuming high quantities of carbohydrates such as: pasta, breads, salted pretzels and chips. Carbohydrates boost our levels of the hormone serotonin, which has a calming effect. This can become a dangerous trap, packing on a lot of pounds quickly.

Nutritional deficiencies that cause cravings

Salt deficiency - Craving for salty snacks. Add Premiers Pink Salt to foods.

Iron deficiency - Craving for red meat is the result of iron deficiency. Instead eating a lot of red meat, eat beans, legumes, dried fruits, spinach, and cherries, and food rich in vitamin C for iron absorption.

Calcium deficiency - Craving for cheese, soda and alcohol. Eat legumes, broccoli, kale, turnip greens, and sesame seeds.

Magnesium deficiency - Craving for sweets (chocolate, acid foods). Substitute chocolate with raw cacao nibs or powder, very dark chocolate, nuts, seeds and fruit.

Phosphorus deficiency - Craving for sweets, coffee or black tea. Eat pumpkin seeds and Brazil nuts, lentils and pinto beans.

Potassium deficiency - Craving for alcohol. Eat citrus fruits, pineapples, bananas, black olives, bitter green leafy vegetables and seaweeds.

Silicone and tyrosine deficiency - Craving for tobacco. Eat nuts, seeds, beetroot, oats, onions, and legumes.

Chromium deficiency - Craving for pasta, white bread, and pastries. Eat apples, cinnamon, romaine lettuce and sweet potatoes.

Nitrogen deficiency - Craving for bread. Eat nuts, grains, legumes and green leafy vegetables.

Chloride deficiency - Craving for potato chips. Eat olives, kelp, tomatoes or celery.

Essential fatty acids deficiency - Craving for potato chips. Eat ground flaxseeds, chia seeds and walnuts.

Stress hormone fluctuations - Craving for popcorn. Eat foods rich in vitamins B and C.

Tyrosine Deficiency - Overeating in general. Eat pumpkin, sesame and sunflower seeds, avocados, bananas, and nuts.

Hormones determine whatever kind of food you eat, and when you eat throughout the day. Different hormones stimulate an appetite for different foods. Refer to the above list to identify your cravings and deficiencies and choose a healthier alternative.

17

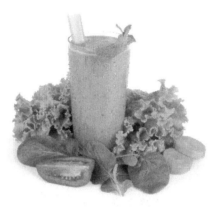

"COME ALIVE" JUICING

Juicing is drinking fresh, nutrient-dense, cold pressed homemade mostly vegetable juices. Juicing is a way to speed up your metabolism and immune system to help you heal from almost every major health challenge you have developed. Juicing places the body in a position to detoxify and let pure antioxidants boost the immune system.

65% of Americans are overweight or obese, and recent data out of John Hopkins University suggests this number will be 75% by 2015. One out of three children born today will develop diabetes. Many of us are low in energy and suffer with chronic pain, and a lack of focus. Our modern diet and lifestyle is to blame.

"If you're green on the inside, you're clean on the inside."

Drinking homemade veggie/fruit juice is low in calories, fat free, and nutrient dense. Fresh juice is very rich in vitamins, minerals, and antioxidants. It is a body boost, giving you energy to help get a better work out. It can also help to suppress your appetite. I add Premiers pink salt to my juice, which helps with digestion, low blood pressure and adrenals. Consuming salt helps keep us hydrated and studies show a deficiency in salt is why some of us reach for the salted potato chips. Believe it or not, having some homemade fresh fruit juice helps control my sugar craving. The other great attribute of consuming homemade raw vegetable juice, is that you feel that energy rush or juice high without the drop of energy that you get after consuming a chocolate bar. Please note that we are talking about homemade mostly vegetable juice, NOT STORE BOUGHT commercial fruit or vegetable juice. Many of those juices contain sugar or corn syrup or are just concentrated fructose, way too much sugar, the same sugar in that candy bar. So don't be fooled. Just Saying!

The Healing Power of Juicing

Juicing is a powerful healing technique that can be used in addition to other therapies to help people heal from pain, cancer, depression, arthritis, severe infections, many autoimmune diseases and other supposedly incurable diseases. The results were nothing short of miraculous. Juicing allows a person to get the maximum amount of nutrition, while still allowing the digestive organs time to rest and heal. A juice fast is a liquid, nourishing, diet consisting of solely vegetable and fruit juices and water. The only restriction for the amount of juice that can be consumed is that you must drink enough juice. In fact, if you drink too little, you will feel hungry, tired, usually gain weight and defeat the healing purpose. When I do a long juice fast, I do not feel hungry at all. I always feel very healthy and you can too if you make sure you get the proper directions. You must be in good health and must drink at least a gallon of fresh raw fruit and vegetable juice daily. You must also have a combination of Premiers supplements, giving you the proper nutrition needed during a long juice fast. This can speed up the benefits of healing tremendously. If you are currently ill, you can do small juice fasts for maybe one, two or three days at a time.

I do suggest a 3 day juice fast to jumpstart your weight loss program, or when you get to a plateau. This is a great way to detox your body, ridding your body of extra toxins it has been holding onto. Always check with your doctor to make sure you are in good health to do a three day juice. Limit your fast to three days, but you can also do it more often.

When juicing, follow these helpful guidelines:

- Vegetables should be as fresh as possible and organic
- Purchase at a local farm when possible
- Use as many leafy greens to enhance healing
- Purchase a juicer (low end - Jack Lalane or Juice Man, or high end - Omega 350)
- Use celery – natures diuretic
- If you make extra juice, pour your juice into wide-mouthed one quart glass mason jars to store for the day (not with low end juicers that incorporate too much oxygen)
- Store your juice in a refrigerator
- Peal all vegetables that are not organic
- Clean all vegetables in limonene or polar mins (from Premier Research Labs)
- Raw juice has beneficial enzymes that give you the nutrients and energy to last throughout the day. I recommend raw juice to everyone, but especially if you are experiencing a time of stress or fatigue. Using a wide variety of vegetables and fruits will expose you to the widest range of minerals and vitamins.

Always use organic for the dirty dozen, and trim the exterior with the clean 15.

Lisa's Favorite Fruit Juice

½ cantaloupe

3 pears

3 oranges

2 red apples

2 green apples

1 lemon

2 cups pineapple

3 cups organic baby carrots

Lisa's Favorite Vegetable Juice

6 large tomatoes

1-2 cloves garlic

6 stalks celery

1 lemon

1 cucumber

1 zucchini

5 kale leaves

1 green pepper

1 red pepper

Banana peppers and Horseradish optional

Add. Pink Salt... Enjoy!

Lisa's Favorite Green Juice
Makes approximately 1 gallon

8 kale leaves

8 large carrots

6 large cucumbers

4 Zucchini

2 inch piece of ginger

6 green apples

3 oranges

1 pack of organic celery

5 lemons

Other Favorites

Organic: Strawberry, apple and pear juice

1 cup organic strawberries, hulls removed

1 organic Granny Smith apple

3 small organic ripe pears

Large bunch of organic Kale

Organic: Carrot, Apple, Kale and Celery juice

3 small organic Granny Smith apples

3 medium sized organic carrots

5 stalks organic celery

Large bunch of organic Kale

1 Lemon (peel off skin)

<u>Organic: Tomato, Cucumber, Kale juice</u>
3 medium organic tomatoes
1 large cucumber, peeled, if not organic
1 large bunch of fresh organic Kale
3 medium organic carrots
1 lemon peeled

Many people do not realize that vegetables contain protein. Here is the amount of protein contained in each vegetable:

<u>Green Vegetables (One cup of the following)</u>
Spinach	3 grams
Watercress	3 grams
Asparagus	3 grams
Broccoli	3 grams
Kale	2.4 grams
Brussels Sprouts	3 grams
*Collard Greens	1 gram

*Good source of vitamin E, protein, omega-3 fatty acids, potassium

Vegetables	Quantity (grams)	Protein Content (grams)
Asparagus	100	3
Aubergine	100	1
Beetroot	100	2
Broccoli	100	3

Brussels Sprouts	100	3
Cabbage	100	1
Carrot	100	0.5
Cauliflower	100	3
Celery	100	0.5
Chicory	100	0.6
Courgette	100	2
Cucumber	100	0.5
Dandelion greens, boiled and without salt	100	2
Endive	100	1
Garlic, raw	100	6
Lentils, boiled and without salt	100	9
Lettuce, green leaf, raw	100	1
Mushrooms, boiled, cooked and drained, without salt	100	2
Marrow	100	0.5
Okra	100	2.43

Onion	100	0.7
Onion Spring	100	2
Pumpkin, cooked, boiled, drained, without salt	100	1
Parsnip	100	1.5
Potato, boiled, without salt	100	2
Radish	100	0.7
Spinach	100	2
Swede	100	0.5
Sweet corn	100	2.5
Squash, boiled and without salt	100	1.64
Sweet potato, cooked, boiled	100	1
Tomato	100	2
Turnip	100	0.8
Watercress	100	3
Yam	100	2

Juicers

I use an Omega 350 Vertical Low Speed Masticating Juicer. The cost is usually around $380 – $425. The Omega's high-speed VRT350 juicer features the superior efficiency of a masticating style juicer in a vertical design. It is compact and productive; this juicer has a processing speed of 80 RPM. An oversized spout makes for easy serving. It weighs only 11 pounds, is stainless steel and easy to clean. The Omega has fine and coarse screens for pulp control; I use the fine screen since I prefer to not have pulp in my juice. The pulp from the juicer is dry meaning it produces a larger yield of juice. This juicer can also handle wheat grass, kale, spinach and collard greens. I make a gallon at a time which takes me an hour to make and clean up, and I can safely store my juice for four to five days. I consume at least a quart of juice a day (when not juice feasting). Make sure if you purchase a juicer you will need to cut up your celery in smaller pieces so it does not clog the juicer, this has come from many, many hours of experience. Also, when juicing softer foods like oranges, follow with something harder like carrots. If the machine stops and is clogged just reverse the on/off button and turn it back on to clear it out.

If you are at all concerned with the oxidation of your juices, or the rate at which they start to break down, it is important to buy a superior juicer over an average one. If you purchase a Jack Lalane or Juiceman, you need to drink the juice immediately after making it. This is due to the oxidation or oxygen exposure. Although I believe a fresh, raw, organic juice is still a power house of nutrition and enzymes, if you are suffering from a complicated health issue and are on a budget, buy the cheaper one and make and drink your juice daily. Oxidation occurs as a result of air (oxygen) exposure, and it begins the process of that food breaking down. A high quality juicer minimizes oxidation. Taking into consideration time requirements, your health realities, and budget, you should be able to feel wonderful about any decision you make with regards to which method you choose to make your juice. Remember, the most important thing is drinking juice. Juice on!

If you can't afford a juicer, then at least take advantage of a blender. Here is the difference between a juicer and a blender. A juicer takes out the fiber and pulp, which would digest into the colon as a normal process of digestion.

However, juice does not digest; it metabolizes immediately, delivering antioxidants directly into the bloodstream. A smoothie made in a blender gives you the bulk needed for healthy digestion. They are both great ways to stay heathy.

"Whole Lot of Shakin Goin On"
Smoothies in a Blender
Celery/Kale/Arugula/Banana

Green smoothies are best made in a powerful blender. Add ½ cup water or half a cup of organic almond milk to the blender, add one stalk celery and one piece of kale. Blend on high for 10 seconds (to a pulp). Then add a pinch of arugula and banana with another ½ cup of almond milk. Add Premiers Greens (1 tbs), Galactin (2 tbs) and Trim Body Whey (4 tbs). Blend and enjoy.

Green Fruit Juice
Apple/Celery/Cucumber/Greens (kale)

Cucumbers mix well with celery in a juice. The organic sodium of the celery helps to transport the water-rich cucumber juice into the tissues, creating more hydration. One of the most beautifying and cleansing of all juices combines celery, apple, and cucumber together.

18

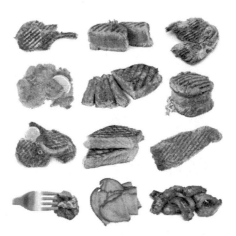

"WE PLUMP WHEN WE COOK IT" EAT RAW, FERMENTED

Cooked food is food that is cooked above 118 degrees for three minutes or longer. When cooked, the protein has become denatured and its sugar has become caramelized, and when the natural fibers have been broken down it is much harder to digest that food. When you eat cooked carbohydrates, proteins, and fats, you are eating numerous (carcinogenic) products caused by the cooking process. If you think of it, we are eating not just dead animals; we are really eating dead meat, lacking anything healthy for us.

Reasons Why You should Not Eat a Lot of Cooked Food

- 80% of the vitamins and minerals are destroyed
- All of the enzymes are completely destroyed
- Pesticides become more toxic, oxygen is lost and free radicals are produced
- Digests in 40 – 100 hours
- Sleepiness after a meal
- Enormous increase of white blood cells (our warriors of defense, our immune system, which come out when we have infection or poisons)
- Quickly ferments and putrefies in the intestinal tract
- Causes allergies hypersensitivities
- Lose up to 97% of the water-soluble vitamins (Vitamins B and C)
- Lose up to 40% of the lipid soluble vitamins (Vitamins A, D, E and K)

"Gnaw on Some Raw"

A *raw food* is a food that is not heated above 118 degrees (F).

- Contains lots of vitamins, minerals, enzymes, a live food
- Digests in 24 – 36 hours
- Raw food provides you with more strength, energy,
- stamina, memory and power of concentration
- Will have energy after a meal
- Usually sleep better
- No increase in white blood cells, which rush in after eating
- Raw foods do not spoil quickly
- Elimination of body odor and halitosis

The Importance of Raw Organic Food for Dogs

My first experience with raw was actually with my dog. I feed my Shelties raw organic chicken and beef. My previous sheltie, Chance, had Lyme disease when he was 1 ½ years old. This compromised his health at a very early age. When he was eight he was diagnosed with cancer. When I first started working for Premier Research Labs, the owner of the company, Dr. Marshall, told me he had raised 50 Shelties on a raw diet for years. Many of his dogs lived to be 20 years old; his oldest lived to be 21. I immediately changed Chance's diet and he lived 5 additional years. He also regained the "pep in his step." I also used Premier supplements to help keep him healthy.

"I Tawt I Taw a Puddy Tat"

But not in this study; all of these cats died out after the third generation. Dr. Francis Pottenger Jr. did an experiment with over 900 cats over a ten year period. The cats were broken into two groups:

Cats fed raw food: a diet of two-thirds raw meat, one-third raw milk, and cod-liver oil.

These cats, were healthy cats, where only 5% developed degenerative diseases or allergies in all four generations.

Cats fed cooked food: a diet of two-thirds cooked meat, one-third raw milk, and cod-liver oil.

1st generation cats – developed degenerative diseases and became lazy in late life.

2nd generation cats – developed degenerative disease by mid- life and lost coordination.

3rd generation cats - developed degenerative diseases (human diseases) very early in life, some were born blind, lived only 6 months, 90% had allergies, skin diseases, parasites, soft bones, and personality disorders.

4th generation cats – all cats died out.

The Milk study

1/3 Raw food with 2/3 raw milk – healthy cats

1/3 Raw food with 2/3 pasteurized, evaporated, condensed milk – cats had health problems similar to the cooked meat study.

After reading the above studies, I certainly believe that raw/live foods are obviously healthier than cooked/dead foods. I think most of you will understand and agree that raw foods are obviously healthier for us, but how many of us can totally convert? This is not necessary, so just add as many live, raw foods into your diet as possible. My diet is mostly raw foods, juice, and some fermented foods. However, I certainly go out to dinner on occasion and enjoy some cooked food. However, as soon as I finish my food, I pop six of Premier's HCL into my mouth. Bottoms up! It is especially important to use HCL when dining out. Many restaurants do not use organic food, and they are not as clean as your kitchen. Don't take the chance, take your HCL.

Cooked foods suppress the immune system and decrease our energy. Think about how you feel after eating a cooked meal. Is it any different than when you eat more raw foods? Your body functions more efficiently when it can digest and absorb your food, delivering the maximum amount of vitamins, minerals and enzymes. The pancreas and liver produce most of the bodies digestive enzymes, so the rest should come from your fresh foods, vegetables, seeds, nuts, sprouted grains, raw milk (if you can tolerate dairy) and enzyme supplements.

If you choose to start on a raw diet, you will notice the weight will start to fly off your body. When you eat raw foods, you will be consuming a large quanity of raw foods since they are very low in calories and high in fiber. When you're not taking in enough sugar from fruit, you'll start craving all sorts of unhealthy foods. Most food lists tell us to limit our fruit intake, don't. When I eat more fruit, it keeps my craving down for the cakes, cookies and donuts that I really want to eat. When you eat fruit, your blood sugar rises and it tells your brain that you are satisfied and you don't crash and burn like you do on the bad stuff; sugar candies, cookies.

"Eat the Best and Leave the Rest"
Organic Fruits

❧ Apple	❧ Dates
❧ Avocado	❧ Lemon
❧ Banana	❧ Lime
❧ Blackberries	❧ Mango
❧ Blueberry	❧ Orange
❧ Cranberries	❧ Papaya

- Raspberry
- Strawberry
- Young coconut

All Organic Vegetables

- Bell peppers: red, orange, yellow
- Broccoli
- Brussel Sprouts
- Cauliflower
- Celery
- Collard Greens
- Garlic
- Ginger
- Jalapeno pepper
- Kale
- Lettuce
- Onion
- Spinach
- Tomato
- Zucchini

Nuts and Seeds

Raw, organic, and preferably soaked then dried in a dehumidifier.

NO PEANUTS

- Almonds
- Brazil
- Cashews
- Filberts
- Macadamia nuts
- Pecans
- Pine nuts
- Pistachio
- Walnuts
- Flax seeds
- Chia seeds
- Hemp seeds
- Sunflower seeds
- Raw almond butter
- Nut "milks"
- Seed crackers (e.g. chia, flax)

Soaked Grains

- Millet
- Buckwheat
- Quinoa
- Oats

Soaked Beans and Legumes/ Organic, Dried, Raw

- Lentils
- Chickpeas
- Adzuki beans
- Mung beans
- Pinto beans

Organic Oil

- Cold-pressed, extra-virgin olive oil
- Raw, virgin coconut oil
- Raw coconut butter
- Chia oil
- Pre-soaked nut butters
- High Quality EFA oil (Premier Research Labs)
- Raw cultured butter

Organic Beverages

- Water
- Vegetable or fruit juice – homemade raw, or organic store bought
- Young coconut water
- Herbal tea (made with water heated to less than 118° F)

Miscellaneous

- Young coconut
- Carob powder
- Raw cacao nibs
- Raw protein powder
- Raw vegan ice cream
- Fermented foods such as miso, kimchee and sauerkraut
- Raw Apple Cider

Herbs, Spices, and Condiments

- Bragg's raw apple cider
- Bragg's liquid aminos
- Cayenne pepper
- Celtic sea salt

- Chocolate, raw
- Cinnamon, ground
- Cumin, ground or seeds
- Curries
- Dill
- Nama shoyu (raw soy sauce)

- Raw honey
- Himalayan salt
- Seaweed
- Sundried tomato
- Vinegars

Sweeteners

- Raw honey
- Agave nectar
- Coconut nectar

- Stevia
- Date sugar
- Yacon

Animal Products

In addition to plant foods, some raw food lists include raw animal foods, such as raw eggs, fish and meat, and non-pasteurized, non-homogenized milk, yogurt and cheese. Consuming raw or undercooked meat, fish, milk, or egg products may increase your risk of foodborne illness. Some people cook the following at a very low temperature, so they are seared on the outside and raw in the middle.

- Fish
- Beef
- Raw Milk

- Raw milk cheese
- Organic egg

Fermented Foods

Fermented foods are all the rage. A fermented food is a food that has had its carbohydrates and sugars turned into alcohol or beneficial acids. They are unpasteurized foods that have gone through a process of fermentation. This fermentation provides a food rich in friendly flora, lactobacilli and enzymes that are extremely beneficial to the entire digestive tract. Our intestinal track contains 80% of our immune system, so it is most important to keep it healthy. When foods are fermented they preserve a healthy living culture important to our digestive system and organ health. Research shows that this process increases the nutrients in the food.

"All things are not created Equal"

Many things are fermented and they are going to be on the *"naughty list,"* don't hate me, coffee, beer, wine, chocolate, sour dough bread, cheese and yogurt. The foods that are on the *"nice list"* are Kiefer, Sauerkraut, Pickles, Kimchi, Kombuchi, Vinegar and Miso.

You can make your own fermented foods, it is so easy, takes only ten minutes and lasts a couple months in the frig. Lacto-fermented foods like this recipe are easier to digest than raw vegetables, and their nutrients are more easily assimilated by our bodies. Plus they are loaded with probiotics that are good for our digestive systems and our overall health.

Making fermented cabbage

Ingredients:

- 1 medium red or green cabbage (about 2 pounds)
- 4 cups water
- 1 tablespoon of our pink salt
- 1 teaspoon caraway seeds, rosemary or garlic (optional)
- 8 to 10 dried juniper berries (optional)

Thinly slice the cabbage into shreds or small pieces. Place in a bowl and mash it for about 4 minutes. Tightly pack the sliced cabbage into clean glass jars, sprinkling in some of the spices or seeds and juniper berries as you fill the clean jars. Make the brine by dissolving the salt in the water. It is important to use non-chlorinated water since chlorine can interfere with the fermentation process. Pour the salt brine over the cabbage and spices when the cabbage is half full. Gently press down on the cabbage and spices very tightly to release any air bubbles. Then add the remaining cabbage, again pressing it down very tightly submerging into the brine. Leave a space of about a half inch at the top of the jar. Leave the jars out at room temperature for 2- 3 days. You should start to see some bubbles on top, which is a sign that fermentation process has started. On the third day put the jars in the refrigerator. The cabbage will have a sour smell and taste. Eat within 3 months. Add to salads or eat it just by itself. Enjoy!

Start out slow if you are not used to eating fermented foods. Start with only one tablespoon and start increasing slowly. A diet rich in raw foods with some fermented foods every day will help to make your body strong and healthy.

19

"I'M LOVIN IT" RELAXATION AND CORTISOL

Cortisol can act as an anti-inflammatory, suppressing the immune system during times of physical and psychological stress. I can't emphasize enough how important it is to practice relaxation to help reduce the cortisol production of belly fat. I was in the hospital for eleven days during my Syringomyelia operation. I noticed after the operation all I wanted to eat was carbs; I pigged out on wheat thins, bagels and even cereal. My diet before the operation included no carbs. While in the hospital I laid in bed all day, beside the occasional walk down the hall with my walker. I was on pain medication which kept me very relaxed and I just watched TV all day. I had bloodwork drawn every day, including the BG/Carb ratio which checked my response to the ingestion of carbohydrates in the form of glucose. What the doctor noticed was upon entering the hospital my carbohydrate level was very low, and the day I left it was very high. She warned me of the dangers of consuming too many carbohydrates, which could raise my blood sugar level. However, I noticed when I returned home I had lost five pounds. Summing up, I ate mostly carbs, got no exercise, relaxed all day and lost five pounds in 11 days. I was blown away. When I got home, I cleaned up my diet, eating no carbs, started walking a mile a day, went back to working on the computer and gained the five pounds back within a week. My only conclusion is that my cortisol levels were so low, it allowed my body to lose weight by just relaxing.

Many systems of bodywork are based on various "energy" models. The Eastern world body therapies are primarily based on the concept of vital life energy chi. The following are a selection of relaxation techniques to add into your life.

"Because You're Worth It" Massage Therapy

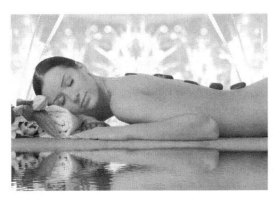

The term bodywork refers to therapies such as massage, deep tissue manipulation, body stretching, which all help to improve the structure and functioning of the human body. Massage helps to promote deep relaxation, reduce pain, soothe injured muscles, and also to stimulate blood and lymphatic circulation. An eastern remedy that has been used for centuries, massage helps to heal the body and reduce tension in everyday life. When people hold tension in their muscles, it contributes to muscle fatigue and pain by compressing the nerve fibers in the muscle and holding in the chemical waste. Massage therapy releases the lactic acid helping the body to detoxify. Also, many people may have neck pain which causes headaches. Massage therapy is a great way to get rid of the constant pain from headaches. It is so important to relieve muscle tension, releasing cortisol, to help you to lose and keep the weight off.

There have been many studies where evidence has supported the benefits of massage therapy. Massage can help muscle spasms, pain, scoliosis, injuries from accidents including whiplash. Lymphatic massage is very helpful in removing toxins from the body, helping to move metabolic wastes through the body and remove toxins to help people recover from illnesses. So reward yourself with a massage instead of food.

"Are you on Pins and Needles?"

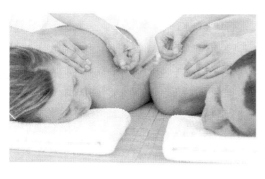

Well you should be. Acupuncture can help you lose weight and to help detox your body. Chinese Acupuncture is four and five thousand years old. Acupuncture and acupressure work on the principle that there are energy channels, called meridians, which run throughout the body. Different organs are associated with different energy meridians, and health problems in various organs show up as energy blocks in the meridians. Acupuncture uses tiny needles to stimulate the flow of Chi or vital energy. They are inserted just under the skin and placed strategically around the body to different acupuncture meridians. The needles are the diameter of three or four strands of hair. Most people find acupuncture to be very relaxing and that it does not hurt. It can remove negative emotions, addictions, stress, body soreness or pain, and almost any disorder or problem that upsets the vitality in the body.

Acupuncture can help with weight loss. Sometimes the body holds in too much heat, which can slow down our metabolism. Acupuncture can help release that heat, helping our bodies to function healthier and shed unwanted pounds. Special acupuncture points are used to help curb food cravings as well. Acupuncture is beneficial in healing conditions with the stomach and digestive track. There are also points that provide a bit of improvement in mood and well-being that would be good for people struggling with weight issues, or who eats to make them feel better. Acupuncture can help with bloating, binge eating, cravings, digestive problems and emotional problems.

Chiropractic

Chiropractic is used by millions to treat back pain. Chiropractors work primarily with the spine, the root of the nervous system through which nerve impulses travel from the brain to the rest of the body. One effect of chronic stress is prolonged muscle tension and contraction. This muscle tension creates uneven pressures on the bony structures of the body, often leading the misalignment of the spinal column, known as subluxations.

Chronic stress also leads to nerve irritation. The adjustments of a chiropractor release muscle tension, which helps the body return to a more balanced, relaxed state. Chiropractic adjustments also reduce spinal nerve irritation, and improve blood circulation. A healthy and balanced spine is one way to effectively manage stress. It helps by developing a healthy response to stress, reducing physical damage which puts stress on the body and causing more cortisol in the body, especially the belly.

Reflexology

Reflexology is a science that deals with the principle that there are reflex areas in the feet and hands, which correspond to all the glands, organs and parts of the body. Reflexology is a soothing technique done by the therapist using pressure points on the foot reflex areas.

Reflexology can relieve tension and stress, improve blood supply, promote the unblocking of energy in your feet, and help your body to achieve balance and harmony.

"The Happiest Place on Earth" Yoga

Relax your mind and body and feel the stress start to dissipate during the first few minutes. Yoga is the practice of body awareness, showing how the mind and body work together. Breathing is the secret to reaching the mind/body connection. As Americans, we live stressful lives and our breathing tends to be very shallow. We tighten up our muscles and somehow forget to relax them. Subsequently, this causes blockages in our bodies, which can lead to disease. In yoga, we learn very deep breathing which conditions body metabolism and lowers our blood pressure and heart rate, stabilizes brain wave frequencies, and causes RELAXATION! Let's not forget that it feels good.

Yoga is a series of different body stretches called postures. Yoga is holistic, meaning it works the whole body. It strengthens and lengthens the muscles in the body, helps eliminate aches and pains, increases your flexibility, and can reverse the aging process. It brings on a feeling of relaxation, balance and clarity. It can make you stronger on the inside and out. Yoga works the following systems: circulatory (blood), respiratory (lungs), endocrine (glands), cardiovascular (heart), muscular system, nervous system, digestion system, skeleton (bones) and articulation (joints). Yoga can strengthen your major muscles (legs, arms, and lower back), minor muscles (wrists, hands and fingers), and organs (heart, lungs, veins, nerves, and tendons).

Yoga is a great place to start, especially if you have not been exercising for a long time. Beginner Yoga classes can be slower and easier to do. It doesn't matter how old or out of shape you are. However, it is always wise to consult a physician if you have any health concerns. Many people feel they need to be flexible before starting a yoga class, when it is actually the opposite. People who start to do yoga will become flexible.

"Make the Most of Now" Meditation

Stay in the moment and learn how to slow down the intense whirlwind of stress by embracing meditation. These skills can weave together your own path to a strong mind/body/spirit connection. Meditation helps us to stay focused and stay in the moment, meaning not dwelling on the past or worrying about the future.

"Yesterday is history, tomorrow is a mystery, and today is a gift, which is why we call it a present"

When I was 13 years old I had the wonderful opportunity of learning from a Maharishi how to do transcendental meditation. I had such a traumatic life filled with stress, that I immediately embraced meditation. In 1970 I met privately with the Maharishi who gave me a mantra, a sound that has no association to a word, to use with my meditation. The first time I meditated I had this sensation in my brain, a release I have never felt before in my life. So, for once, I was hooked on "a good thing" early in my life.

Meditation is a safe and simple way to balance a person's physical, emotional, and mental states. It is easily learned and has been used as an aid in treating stress, pain management, hypertension and heart disease. Meditation has been practiced for several thousand years. Today, the science of meditation proves through extensive studies that the frontal lobe of the brain goes offline, the thalamus reduces the flow of incoming information to a trickle, and the parietal lobe slows down. Studies have shown that a person that meditates actually has lower blood pressure, uses 17% less oxygen, lowered heart rates by three beats a minute and increases their theta brain waves (the ones that appear right before sleep).

The purpose of meditation is to make our mind calm and peaceful. People who meditate find that they worry less and are much more peaceful and happy. Meditation does not have to be complex. It tones and tunes up the thinking processes and the emotions and brings everyday life into sharper focus with new degrees of ease and harmony. Meditation requires nothing on your part but the time it takes to do it.

There are so many types of meditation. There are Breath Meditations, Transcendental Meditation (TM) mantra meditations, walking meditations, and guided meditations. All meditations have a few things in common; we need to focus on something such as a word, mantra (sound), ocean waves or breath. Then when our mind starts to wander we slowly come back to our breath or sound. When using a mantra, we come back by thinking of that sound over and over. During meditation, we try to ignore all of the distractions around us; noise in our head, talking, cars outside, or even a clock. As we become more advanced, we can meditate and not even hear the distractions.

It is best not to eat before meditation, but if you are really hungry try a nutrition bar or piece of fruit. When meditating at home, try to create a peaceful atmosphere by disconnecting your phone, closing your door for privacy, and putting any animals out of the room.

Let's try a little meditation.

1. Find a quiet place, turn out the lights, sit comfortably in a chair, lying is not recommended since many people tend to fall asleep instead of meditating.
2. Close your eyes and shut out the world; begin to relax the muscles in your body.
3. Next breathe naturally, preferably through the nostrils inhaling and exhaling.
4. Just continue to follow your breath, becoming aware of the sensation of the breath as it enters and leaves the nostrils. If you prefer to use a sound, you can use the universal sound of "om" as your mantra.
5. At first our mind will be very busy and we might think that mediation is making our mind busier, but we are really just becoming more aware of how busy our mind is. Thoughts and distractions, including worries, our kids, things we need to be doing, disagreements with friends, and noises outside will enter our mind. Once we realize that we are distracting, we can gently bring ourselves back to the meditation and start to follow our breath or repeat the "om" sound silently. The more we practice, the more patient and relaxed we will become. Our mind will feel clear and spacious and refreshed. Eventually thinking less about our distractions.
6. I usually practice meditation for twenty minutes daily. It is best to start out small and work up to longer sessions. It is recommended to meditate twice a day, once in the morning and again in the early evening.

20

"BET YOU CAN'T EAT JUST ONE" LEGAL DRUGS

Did you EVER hear of someone healing from Heart disease or Diabetes from taking medications? People on medications will take their medications to their grave. Medical doctors learn in medical school how to do surgery, remove organs and to prescribe medications. Medications are only a Band-Aid, a temporary way to treat only symptoms and relieve pain. However, medical doctors are essential for life threatening accidents and all acute situations. The medical doctors treat the symptoms, not cure the problem. If you get an UTI, you take an antibiotic, which will get rid of the infection only temporarily. Most people will then get the same infection again. Why? The toxicity will come out in different locations in the body, or different organs, most likely where an organ is more deficient or toxic. Remember the original problem still has not been addressed. People will need to detox their bodies with supplements, improve their diets and detox those organs that are toxic.

Are the medications you are taking making you worse? Did you know that alcohol is a drug? "Say no to drugs," Users are losers," there is no difference between illicit drugs and prescription drugs. Medications lower your pH even more because they are on the acid side of the food and drug charts. They make your immune system even more depressed, causing more internal infections, squashing your energy and making your body even weaker. The greatest cause of death, following a successful surgery is secondary infection. With a depressed immune system, secondary infections are deadly. The danger is that almost all medications are used forever/permanently and they are altering and changing your body's natural functions. *"Riddle Me This"* Has your doctor ever taught you how to live healthy?

If you are currently taking any type of medication, never detox yourself. Instead make an appointment with your doctor to follow the proper instructions for your detox. I recommend healing your body first with the life changing therapies in this book before you ever think of getting off of your medications. Most of you will heal and the proof with be the blood test results from your doctor telling you that you no longer need medication. Insert, Happy Dance!

How did I get sick? *"Let me count the ways"*

Smoking, medications, drugs & alcohol, stress, surgeries, bad teeth (infection and mercury fillings), poor mental health, eating meats & dairy products with (steroids, pesticides and antibiotics), eating junk foods, eating sugar, eating out often, eating fast food, white flour products, and drinking caffeine (coffee & sodas) are just a few ways we abuse our bodies daily. "If you continue to do what you have always done, you will continue to develop what you have created." POOR HEALTH!

Prescription medication is part of daily life for millions of people worldwide. In fact most people put all of their trust in their medical doctors, to lead them down the path to health. It has been stated that when medications are used in accordance with medical guidelines, they can maintain health and sustain life. This is true, but nothing is stated about healing from these diseases or disorders. It is not just prescription medications that are abused; many illegal drugs such as cocaine, amphetamines and heroin and many legal drugs such as alcohol and nicotine.

Over 100,000 people die each year from prescription drug side effects in the U.S. alone. This does NOT include deaths from doctors accidentally prescribing the wrong drugs, nor from pharmacists filling the prescription incorrectly, nor from patients overdosing. Researchers have estimated that medications cause 17 million visits to emergency rooms and 8.7 million hospitalizations each year. Medicines are one of the leading causes of death in America, it becomes imperative for physicians, pharmacists and patients to be aware of those drugs that are most likely to cause problems and in certain circumstances even death.

Drugging America – The Big Bucks

Washington D.C., March 27, 2011 – Pharmaceuticals are a $650 plus billion dollar a year industry. For years the most profitable business in the U.S. has been the pharmaceutical corporations, which routinely top the annual fortune 500 list. Doctor's prescribe drugs to support an industry, which out-earns the Gross National Product, (GNP) of many nations.

A new study from York University on January 7, 2008 "estimates the U.S. pharmaceutical industry spends almost twice as much on promotion as it does on research and development, contrary to the industry's claim. The U.S. pharmaceutical industry spent 24.4% of the sales dollar in 2004 on promotion, versus 13.4% for research and development, as a percentage of US domestic sales of US $235.4 billion."

Why are they advertising Drugs on Television?

Why are they? Did you know that drug companies spend over 5 billion dollars in drug advertising a year? When advertising a product the ultimate purpose is for that item to make money. The pharmaceutical companies are so "in our faces," and their drug sales and profits are up. The drugs may be legal, but the drugs do the same thing to your body that the illegal drugs do, they lower your immune system. Sure people are living longer, but with what quality of life.

The following are the trusted legal drugs, common prescription medications that are harmful when used Chemotherapy Drugs

Chemotherapy drugs, such as methotrexate, are actually poisons that are prescribed to kill cancer cells in the body and are the number one most toxic drug on the market. These drugs also kill healthy cells in the body. Chemotherapeutic agents are also prescribed to treat ailments such as rheumatoid arthritis. Health risks associated with extended use of chemotherapeutic agents are death, congenital abnormalities, liver toxicity, kidney toxicity, lung disease, bone marrow loss, internal bleeding, ulceration and suppressed immune system. There are many theories out there, but many agree that it is not the cancer that is killing people; it is the chemotherapy that is poisoning their bodies.

Prednisone

Millions of people are taking prednisone, the corticosteroid drug that is widely prescribed for conditions such as asthma, emphysema, allergies, Crohn's disease, Multiple Sclerosis, herniated spinal discs, acute muscular pain syndromes, Type 2 Diabetes, Rheumatoid Arthritis, intestinal bleeding, autoimmune diseases, and to reduce inflammation from a variety of medical problems. Prednisone is meant to be a short-term medication and can be very dangerous if used long-term. Long term side effects include high blood pressure, fluid retention, potassium loss, muscle weakness, osteoporosis, fracture of long bones and broken vertebrae, peptic ulcers, intestinal bleeding, and much more. This is considered one of the most dangerous medications in the pharmaceutical line up.

Blood Thinners

Blood thinning agents such as Coumadin (warfarin) are commonly prescribed to prevent strokes and heart attacks. Individuals taking these types of medication should use extreme caution since severe bleeding can result even from the smallest cut or scratch. Death can result from excessive blood loss from what would seem to be a minor injury in individuals taking this type of medication.

Dr. Daniel Budnitz and his colleagues at the Centers for Disease Control and Prevention (CDC) analyzed data from 58 hospitals that participated in an adverse drug-event surveillance project. The researchers were looking for medications that led to emergency hospitalizations. They found that blood thinners were especially problematic. Roughly one-third of all the admissions were from warfarin (Coumadin). Clinical trials have proven that all rats and mice die when they ingest enough Coumadin or Warfarin...they bleed to death!

Prozac

Prozac (fluoxetine) is a medication prescribed to 6 million Americans for depression which alters the mechanism that balances levels of serotonin in the brain. High levels of serotonin in the brain can cause agitation and anxiety, while low levels can cause depression. Drugs such as Prozac can cause constant agitation and suicidal thoughts, hostility and violent behavior. Did you know that students involved in the school shooting such as Columbine, the Stock Trading Center and the Jewish Daycare Center were all on either, Prozac, Zoloft or Ritalin? There are so many things that cause depression other than a loss from death or a relationship such as medical depression from sickness, deficiencies in Vitamin B complex, too many carbohydrates, alcohol, tobacco and so much more. Changing your diet and adding many super antioxidants can help low grade depression without medication.

ADD/ADHD Medication

Ritalin and Adderall are medications used to treat conditions like Attention Deficit Disorder (ADD) and Attention Deficit Hyperactivity Disorder ADHD. These are amphetamines and their main purpose is to speed up the body making it easier to focus. These drugs are highly addictive and cause side effects such as anxiety, hostility, exhaustion, and trouble sleeping. Many doctors will then give children a sleeping pill to help the insomnia. This breaks my heart that doctors that we trust would start young children on these drugs, setting them up for such an unhealthy life and addiction. These medications are very over prescribed.

"To Heal or To Medicate -That is the Question!"

You have to ask yourself, do I give my child a pill and try and make it all go away, or do I invest the time and re-evaluate the foods our family eats and try to make a change there. Below are suggestions that are mostly diet related, to help with ADD and ADHD.

A good night's sleep is essential, in addition your child needs to be outside in the sun every day, use Premiers Pink Salt (1/2 tsp a day), exercise and drink plenty of water. Then you need to eliminate all junk food, fast food, white flour, MSG, and processed foods then start consuming sulfur foods from the list below:

Sulfur Foods

- Garlic, onions, and all of the allium family
- Grains: Oats
- Methionine: sunflower seeds, oats, dark chocolate, cashews, walnuts, almonds, sesame seeds (in that order)
- cysteine: oats
- Legumes, including carob and jicama (alfalfa MSM)
- Eggs – chicken and duck eggs
- Nuts & seeds
- Broccoli, all cruciferous vegetables, cabbages, pak choi, mustard, and watercress
- Asparagus
- Coconut
- Avocado
- Watermelon (glutathione)
- Swiss Chard
- Parsley
- Sweet potatoes and yams
- Bananas
- Tomatoes (MSM)
- Tea (MSM)
- Whey proteins (high in cysteine & methionine)
- Amino acids: cysteine, methionine

Note: Methylsulfonylmethane (MSM) helps to reduce histamine in your body, which is the inflammatory substance responsible for many allergy symptoms.

Supplements

- B Complex
- Magnesium

- Vitamin D
- DHA
- Zinc

Also many studies show that a Gluten Free diet can help ADD and ADHD kids and adults.

Pain Killers

The 4th leading cause of death in the United States is from pain medications. Millions of people take some form of pain medication every single day. They are very addictive and have the longest and most severe detox symptoms of most drugs. They are also used to relieve discomfort/pain from an injury, surgery or disease. Over 15,000 people die annually from overdosing on opiate pain medications which is more than heroin and cocaine deaths combined. There are many types of pain medications including:

- Nonsteroidal anti-inflammatory drugs (NSAIDs)
- Corticosteroids which are often administered as an injection at the site of musculoskeletal injuries. Acetaminophen increases the body's pain threshold, but it has little effect on inflammation.
- Opioids/Opiates - Codeine, Morphine, Hydrocodone, Vicodin, and Oxycodone modify pain messages in the brain.
- Muscle relaxants – Flexeril and Valium reduce pain from tense muscle groups, most likely through sedative action in the central nervous system.

Natural Therapies to help with pain – Massage, Chiropractic, Acupuncture, Reiki, Premiers Deltanol-Deltatocotrienol form of vitamin E, (similar to the mechanism of Ibuprofen.)

Diuretics

As a diet addict, I loved using my diuretics because I could shed 5 pounds in a couple hours which would be the deciding factor if I would or would not fit into my jeans. When you think about that, you can see how dangerous that is. Physicians are ready to prescribe diuretics to lower hypertension. They may lower blood pressure but they also rid your body of many essential minerals such as potassium, sodium, chloride, zinc and iodine, calcium, and magnesium. Diuretics are very dangerous and contribute to thousands of deaths per year. The loss of these minerals can lead to stroke, irregular heart rhythms and heart attack.

Holistic Alternatives would include RenaVen (kidney support), UriVen (bladder support) and ImmunoND (to open up lymphatic drainage). Make sure to drink plenty of filtered water every day.

Statins for Cholesterol Reduction

Cholesterol medications called statins include Mevacor, Zocor and Pravachol, just to name a few. Statins are used to reduce cholesterol production in the liver and change the method in which LDL cholesterol enters the cells. Statin drugs can have some of the following side effects: headache, inflammation, joint and muscle pain, burning or painful urination; and lower back and side pain. People taking statin drugs, need to have annual liver function tests.

"Make up Your Mind"

Why is it that the numbers keep being lowered for those who need cholesterol medication? Over the years, blood test results for cholesterol levels have been lowered from 359 to the current level of 200. "According to Lynn Payer, in her book *Medicine and Culture*, the median total cholesterol range for initiating drug therapy was 340 to 359 mg/dl in 1983, 300 to 319 in 1986, 240 to 259 in 1990, and that same year dietary therapy was instituted at levels of 200 to 219 mg/dl total serum cholesterol."

Holistic approach: Many people can reduce their cholesterol by changing and cleaning up their diets, choosing healthy fats, increased fiber with fruits and vegetables, taking vitamins E, C, Folic Acid and B vitamins and eliminating fatty fried foods.

Nonsteroidal anti-inflammatory drugs (NSAID) We are all familiar with over the counter medications Aleve, Motrin and Ibuprofen. We use them for pain relief for headaches, colds and body aches. They are the most prescribed medications for treating conditions such as arthritis. Did you know they account for approximately 16,000 deaths per year?

Diabetes Drugs

I had Type 2 Diabetes for about a year. Blood sugar levels should normally be at 80 to 120 upon waking up and before meals. My blood sugar test revealed that my sugar reading was usually 175. However, my diabetes was not related to food. I had adrenal fatigue at the time and my diet was almost perfect. Once I added mud pack detoxing and started taking the correct supplements, my Type 2 Diabetes disappeared and has not returned. Type 2 Diabetes, or non-insulin dependent diabetes, is the most common form of diabetes. Medications such as Glucotrol, Tolinase and Micronase are often prescribed to control it. This has side effects such as hypoglycemia, headaches, gastrointestinal problems, fatigue and liver damage. One of the warnings for these prescriptions is the increase in deaths from heart attacks. If someone tells you Diabetes is genetic, please do some research. Diabetes today is so prevalent; if it was genetic then why has the increase been so dramatic in the last 15 years? Do your homework and you will see that a diet high in sugar, fast foods, carbs and processed foods is the culprit.

Healthy Prescription: Reduce/Eliminate your alcohol, carbohydrates, and sugar consumption and add in healthy proteins, fruits and vegetables to eliminate your Diabetes. Exercise on a daily basis. Use RenaVen for kidney strength to help prevent excessive urination and Premiers PancroVen for healthy blood sugar.

Arthritis Drugs

More than 37 million people are afflicted with arthritis. Many people use Motrin, where others use prescriptions such as Celebrex, Ansaid, Clinoril, Vicodin and Naproxen. These drugs take care of the symptoms and the pain; however pain is our body's indication that something is wrong. The side effects include the destruction of cartilage lining at the end of bones.

Holistic Approach for Arthritis – Deltinol to reduce inflammation, NucleoVen or Allicidin for mycoplasma infection and Osteoven to supply calcium and Vitamin D, Turmeric, Liver ND, Gallbladder ND, Hepatoven, and Biliven.

Beta Blockers

Beta blockers are a class of drugs prescribed to lower blood pressure. Beta blockers include Inderal, Tenormin, Lopressor, Corgard and Normodyne. These medications alter the heart's ability to respond to stimulators such as adrenaline and epinephrine. In addition they compromise the function of the heart to weaken it and relax the blood vessels so blood pressure is lowered and heart pain is reduced. This class of medication also causes some serious side effects such as loss of libido, impotence, elevated blood lipids and compromised cardiac function. The Physician's Desk Reference clearly warns physicians of the dangers of long term use of beta blockers: shortness of breath, cold extremities, palpitations, congestive heart failure and hypertension.

High Blood Pressure

Diuretics, alpha and beta blockers, ACE Inhibitors, calcium channel blockers, and blood vessel dilators are used to lower the blood pressure. Many have been linked with serious risks for such conditions as different types of cancer, heart attack, liver damage and stroke.

Many researchers are convinced that using these drugs to treat high blood pressure has played a major role in the epidemic of congestive heart failure in the United States. In 1979 there were 377,000 hospitalizations for congestive heart failure. Only 12 years later, that number had risen to 822,000.

Holistic Solution: Use healthy fats such as raw nuts, avocados, and olive oils, use pink sea salt, exercise, stress reduction such as yoga, meditation and massage.

Proscar

Proscar is used to shrink an enlarged prostate. It may provide benefits such as decreased urge to urinate, better urine flow with less straining, less of a feeling that the bladder is not completely emptied, and decreased nighttime urination. It is not approved for the prevention of prostate cancer, in fact it may slightly increase the risk of developing a very serious form of prostate cancer. 40,000 men a year die from prostate cancer.

Holistic Help: Use Premiers: ProstaVen and Testosterone

Alcohol

Alcohol is one of the most dangerous and accessible drugs available. Alcohol is highly addictive and has very hard and dangerous detox symptoms. Although many people drink alcohol socially, it is a poison for the body, especially the liver. The number of alcoholic liver disease deaths is 16,749 and the number of alcohol-induced deaths, excluding accidents and homicides, is 26,654. You should limit or eliminate alcohol completely. If you are drinking alcohol, make sure you know that it takes 24 hours for your liver to process the alcohol from your body. If you drink daily, the alcohol will eventually cause cirrhosis of the liver or other complications.

21

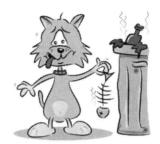

"DON'T MAKE A RUN FOR THE BORDER" TOXINS, WHAT'S SAFE?

Fishy, Fishy

The Institute for Health and the Environment at the University of Albany found that farmed salmon contain potentially harmful levels of PCB's, dioxins, dieldrin and toxaphene. The levels of contamination in the farmed salmon were as much as **10 times that found in the wild salmon.** "Now, will that get you to pay more for wild caught fish?" I hope so; your health is worth it.

The following is a quote from the FDA's website.

"How do drug residues end up in fish? Some fish are given drugs to treat bacterial and parasitic diseases that cause major mortalities in fish. The FDA's

Center for Veterinary Medicine (CVM) regulates drugs given to animals. CVM conducts research to improve the drug approval process and expand the number of safe drugs available for fish production. CVM also develops methods to detect unapproved chemicals in fish tissues so that harmful drug residues don't wind up in the fish on your plate."

"It's safe until proven otherwise" Wrong

What Is Dioxin?

Dioxin is the name generally given to a class of super-toxic chemicals, the chlorinated dioxins and furans, formed as a by-product of the manufacture, molding, or burning of organic chemicals and plastics that contain chlorine. It is the nastiest, most toxic man-made organic chemical; its toxicity is second only to radioactive waste. The major sources of dioxin are in our diet. Dioxin is fat-soluble, 97.5% is found in meat and dairy products. If you are eating the typical American diet, you get the most dioxin from beef, chicken, pork, fish, dairy products, milk and eggs, in that order.

How to Avoid Dioxin

Do not eat beef or pork unless it is organic. Limit your intake of ocean fish; do not eat any freshwater fish. Chicken has the lowest dioxin content of all meats, but is still significant. Vegetarian meat substitutes such as tofu, beans, and rice have essentially no dioxin contamination. If your family drinks milk or eats cheese, use only organic dairy products.

An organic compound is any member of a large class of gaseous, liquid, or solid chemical compounds whose molecules contain carbon. Avoid all organic chemicals that have "chloro" as part of their names such as:

- Wood preservative pentachlorophenol
- Chlorine bleach (Use oxygen bleach instead)
- Use unbleached paper products
- Weed killers and insecticides
- Permethrin flea sprays for pets
- Household toys packaged in polyvinyl chloride

- Saran Wrap unless identified as polyethylene
- Cottonseed oil in (potato chips)
- Cotton sprayed with chlorophenol insecticides
- Soaps made with tallow (made from animal fat)
- Deodorant soaps and deodorants with triclosan, a Chlorophenol
- Chlorine bleached coffee filters
- Wash fruits and vegetables to remove chlorophenol pesticide
- residue (no grapes or raisins)

"Rescuing Good Health from Bad Science" GMO

A genetically modified organism (GMO) is an organism whose genetic material has been altered, where plants or animals are created through the gene splicing techniques of biotechnology. Organisms that have been genetically modified include micro-organisms such as bacteria and yeast, insects, plants, fish, and mammals. This experimental technology merges DNA from different species, creating unstable combinations of plant, animal, bacterial and viral genes that cannot occur in nature or in traditional crossbreeding. Many herbicide resistant corn and soybean varieties have been engineered over the past 15 to 20 years. These include varieties with resistance to the herbicide glyphosate (the active ingredient in Roundup®).

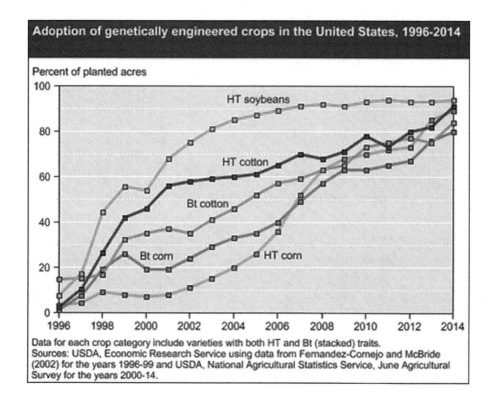

Adoption of genetically engineered crops in the United States, 1996-2014

Percent of planted acres

Data for each crop category include varieties with both HT and Bt (stacked) traits.
Sources: USDA, Economic Research Service using data from Fernandez-Cornejo and McBride
(2002) for the years 1996-99 and USDA, National Agricultural Statistics Service, June Agricultural
Survey for the years 2000-14.

The above graph shows the increase in GMO produced foods. This is unacceptable. Remember, organic is non GMO. Protect yourself from this dangerous process and pesticide use.

Below is a list of foods that are most contaminated or have risky ingredients. It is to your advantage that you stay away from these products as well.

High-Risk Crops (in commercial production; ingredients derived from these must be tested every time, prior to use, in Non-GMO Project Verified products (as of December 2011):

- Alfalfa (first planting 2011)
- Canola (approx. 90% of U.S. crop)
- Corn (approx. 88% of U.S. crop in 2011)
- Cotton (approx. 90% of U.S. crop in 2011)

- Papaya (most of Hawaiian crop; approximately 988 acres)
- Soy (approx. 94% of U.S. crop in 2011)
- Sugar Beets (approx. 95% of U.S. crop in 2010)
- Zucchini and Yellow Summer Squash (approx. 25,000 acres)

Lower Risk

- Tomatoes
- Potatoes

Hormone Drugs - Serving Poison on Your Dinner Plate

It is a sin to see how cruel animals are treated today. Meat is chemically injected with more and more toxins, forcing the size of the animal growth to *"plump up the volume."* It is becoming harder and harder to eat healthy. Here's how it works: hormone drugs are manufactured as a pellet and are put under the skin of the animal's ear and discarded when they are slaughtered. It is hard to believe, that in the U.S., all of the steroid hormone growth-promoting drugs are available as over-the-counter purchases. There are 6 FDA approved hormones, 3 synthetic and 3 natural, for use in the beef industry. The 3 synthetic ones are melengestrol acetate, trenbolone acetate and zeranol and the 3 natural ones are estradiol, progesterone and testosterone. There are nearly 3,000 chemical additives which are approved for use in food. Yikes!

Most traditionally raised beef calves go from 80 pounds to 1,200 pounds in a period of about 14 months. Wow that's fast! Today's cows are fed high quantities of corn and implanted with different drugs to fatten them up quickly.

Meat producers poison the animal from birth to death and you serve these chemicals to your family, your children's health is especially at risk. Some producers are now injecting the slaughtered meat with water, sodium phosphate and sodium to add tenderness and weight. There is no reason to buy **NON**-organic meat.

Measurable amounts of hormones in traditionally raised beef are transferred to humans, and some scientists believe that human consumption of estrogen from hormone-fed beef can result in cancer, premature puberty and falling sperm counts.

I hypothesize that there are many adults and children that consume more than 50% of their diets eating very high quantities of non-organic meats, milk and cheese. At what point do we call this safe consumption, when ingesting such high levels of hormones while eating high amounts of daily protein. The more we eat, the more chemicals we ingest...right? I was not able to find many studies on hormones in protein in the U.S. and the effects it has had on us for cancers and early puberty in girls. Why? What are they afraid they will find?

Ganmaa Davaasambuu is a physician (Mongolia), a Ph.D. in environmental health (Japan), a fellow (Radcliffe Institute for Advanced Study), and a working scientist (Harvard School of Public Health). Her studies have led her to be suspicious in the role cow milk, cheese and other dairy products play in the hormone cancers including prostate, testes and breast. The link between cancer and dietary hormones, estrogen in particular, has been a source of great concern among scientists, said Ganmaa, but it has not been widely studied or discussed. She feels the potential risk is large. Natural estrogens are up to 100,000 times more potent than their environmental counterparts, such as the estrogen-like compounds in pesticides."

Ganmas is quoted as saying "Among the routes of human exposure to estrogens, we are mostly concerned about cow's milk, which contains considerable amounts of female sex hormones. Part of the problem seems to be milk from modern dairy farms where cows are milked about 300 days a year. For much of that time, the cows are pregnant. The later in pregnancy a cow is the more hormones appear in her milk. Milk from a cow in the late stage of pregnancy contains up to 33 times as much of a signature estrogen compound (estrone sulfate) than milk from a non-pregnant cow and 10 times more progesterone than raw."

Butter, meat, eggs, milk, and cheese are implicated in higher rates of hormone-dependent cancers in general, she said. Breast cancer has been linked particularly to consumption of milk and cheese. In another study, rats fed milk show a higher incidence of cancer and develop a higher number of tumors than those who drank water, said Ganmaa.

Antibiotics In Meats: The truth is you are eating sick animals

From birth to slaughter, animals in production feed lots and all non-organic production sites, are given antibiotics constantly whether they are sick or not. This is done because these animals are raised in small cages, fed corn (makes animals sick) and some never see the light of day. Infections run rampant because of the overcrowding and dirty facilities. We already know that toxins are living in our organs, but many believe these hormones cause a host of problems for young girls reproductively. Every time you drink non-organic milk or eat non-organic meat, you are dosing yourself with a constant supply of antibiotics. What this means is that people are becoming more and more resistant to antibiotics, meaning you may need a stronger antibiotic when you do get sick.

FDA Wants Voluntary Decrease of Antibiotics Used
Do You Think This Will Work?

The FDA revealed that sales of the two most commonly used antibiotics in livestock and poultry increased for the second consecutive year. Ranchers purchased 14.4 million pounds of penicillin and tetracycline in 2011, a 2.9 million pound increase from 2009. The U.S. Food and Drug Administration announced that they are "taking three steps to protect public health and promote the judicious use of medically important antibiotics in food-producing animals." The FDA issued a voluntary initiative to make some changes by issuing three documents that will help veterinarians, farmers and animal producers by limiting their antibiotic use to only address disease and health problems. If you voluntarily asked doctors to limit the use of drugs to patients do you think they would?

Organic Free Roaming - What's the difference

Organic free roaming outdoor animals have much stronger immune systems and seldom get sick. However, if one does get sick they are removed from the herd permanently if given antibiotics. Certified organic meats will not contain any antibiotics.

Animals raised for the purpose of providing certified organic meats are not allowed to eat any food which has been treated with synthetic fertilizers, pesticides, herbicides, sewage sludge or radiation. Their food sources cannot contain any preservatives, additives or GMO's. Organic grass fed cows are an excellent source of conjugated linoleic acid (CLA) and the meat is leaner, and has a better fatty acid ratio. Research has found that raw dairy products and meat from grass fed cattle can have CLA levels at 30% to 50% higher than those of cattle fed a diet of primarily corn and grain. CLA has been found to reduce body fat, especially abdominal fat, combat Arteriosclerosis and help fight the onset of diabetes. CLA was found to improve insulin levels in about two-thirds of diabetic patients, and moderately reduced the blood glucose level and triglyceride levels. CLA reduces fat and preserves muscle tissue.

"We Don't Do Chickens Right"

The FDA has admitted some of chicken meat sold in the USA contains arsenic, a cancer-causing toxic chemical. The move follows a recent FDA study of 100 broiler chickens that detected inorganic arsenic, a known carcinogen, at higher levels in the livers of chickens treated with 3-Nitro, compared with untreated chickens. The U.S. Food and Drug Administration recently announced that Alpharma, a subsidiary of Pfizer Inc., will voluntarily suspend U.S. sales of the animal drug 3- Nitro (Roxarsone). American consumers who eat conventional chicken have been swallowing arsenic, a known cancer-causing chemical since 1940.

White Rice

FDA has increased its testing of rice and rice products to determine the level and types of arsenic found in these products. "On September 6, 2013, the FDA released the results of approximately 1,300 samples of rice and rice products examined for the presence of arsenic. The announcement followed the release in September 2012 of a preliminary set of analytical results of nearly 200 samples of rice products tested for arsenic. Taken together, these approximately 1,300 samples comprise the largest data set available on arsenic in rice and rice products."

The United Kingdom and India published a study providing the first evidence that eating rice with high levels of arsenic can lead to genetic damage in cells associated with cancer. Elevated amounts of arsenic in rice can cause genetic damage in people who consume this staple food.

Sugar

Too much sugar isn't good for anyone, especially when it is stripped of all its minerals. Frequently, companies are using genetically modified sugar beets to make sugar found in drinks. This can overload your liver, decay teeth, cause insulin resistance which can lead to Type 2 diabetes. Sugar is also highly addictive.

Dextrose

Dextrose (also known as glucose) is used in medical applications when a patient is unable to consume enough liquids. It is also used as an artificial sweetener in foods. Excessive use of dextrose been linked to obesity, diabetes, high blood sugar (hyperglycemia) and lack of sodium in the blood.

Citric acid

Citric acid is used as a preservative, as well as an acidic or sour taste in foods. It can actually be harmful if you have a history of electrolyte/mineral imbalances. MSG has been found in some citric acid.

Monosodium Glutamate (MSG)

MSG is a chemical flavor enhancer that is used to cover up old stale tastes that you would not normally eat. Many people have allergies and cannot tolerate MSG. Our government allows MSG to be secretly included in many products under hidden names such as "natural flavors", spices, broth, HVP and many more. MSG is included in many products including meats, crackers, bread, candy, chips, fruit juices, salad dressing and canned items. Symptoms include bloating, headaches/migraines, skin rashes, nausea, sweating, chest pain and back pain, etc. Stay away from all processed prepared foods and ask when you are purchasing Chinese food to see if it contains MSG.

Natural Flavor

Natural flavor is anything but natural and it is usually not good for you. The substance is extracted, then chemically altered to taste like it would have before it was modified.

Under the Code of Federal Regulations, the definition for natural flavor is: "the essential oil, oleoresin, essence or extractive, protein hydrolysate, distillate, or any product of roasting, heating or enzymolysis, which contains the flavoring constituents derived from a spice, fruit or fruit juice, vegetable or vegetable juice, edible yeast, herb, bark, bud, root, leaf or similar plant material, meat, seafood, poultry, eggs, dairy products, or fermentation products thereof, whose significant function in food is flavoring rather than nutritional" (21CFR101.22).

Salt

Salt is extremely dangerous for many people. In its natural state is a brown color so it is chemically cleaned with aluminum, ferroancyanide and bleach, to make it a more pleasant white color. This process removes all nutrients and minerals.

Sodium Citrate

Sodium Citrate is the sodium salt of citric acid. Gives drinks their salty and sour taste. It is can be used to regulate acid in drinks. Side effects include nausea, stomach ache, loose stools, and vomiting.

Monopotassium Phosphate

Monopotassium phosphate is a source of potassium that is used as a food additive to emulsify oils that would otherwise separate. It also acts as a thickener, acidity regulator and stabilizer, fertilizer and fungicide.

Yellow 6

Yellow 6 food dye has been linked to learning and concentration disorders in children. It can aggravate ADHD symptoms. There are also animal studies that have shown a potential risk for tumors in kidneys and intestinal areas.

Tobacco

We all know that smoking is dangerous even if you are just around someone that smokes. Cigarettes contain Benzene, which is found in gasoline, formalde-hyde, pesticides, and Tobacco-specific N-nitrosamines (TSNAs).

Bread

Today, flour contains sodium diacetate to inhibit mold, monoglycerides, potassium bromate, aluminum phosphate, calcium phosphate monobasic, chloromine T (as a bleach) and aluminum potassium sulfate. Look at all the chemicals...why? All the more reasons to...Buy Organic!

Butter

Butter has hydrogen peroxide as a bleaching agent, yellow No. 3 coloring and nordihydroguaiaretic acid as an antioxidant. Again...Buy Organic!

Milk

Non-organic milk contains hydrogen peroxide, oat gum, antibiotics, fungicides, pesticides and hormones. In addition to milk, make sure you purchase all of your cheese, cottage cheese, yogurt and all other dairy under the organic label. Buy Organic! Seeing a trend yet?

Canned foods

Can you pronounce all of these? If you can't, know they are chemicals. Real organic natural products are going to have simple ingredients. Canned foods contain: sorbic acid (fungistate), Butylated hydroxyanisole, Mono- and di-glycerides, Poly oxyethylene (20), sorbitan monolaurate (flavor dispersant),

Sodium alginate, Calcium carbonate, Cinnamaldehyde Titanimoxide, Mannitol, Petrolatum (candy polish), Propyleneglycol (mold inhibitor), Calcium oxide, Sodium citrate, and Sodium benzoate, just to name a few.

Simply put, do not use canned foods.

Almond Milk

Almond milk contains sodium carbonate which can be dangerous to the gastro-intestinal track. Effects can include hoarseness, throat swelling, difficulty swallowing, drooling, vomiting, diarrhea, and severe pain in the mouth, throat, chest and abdomen, rapid and life-threatening drop in blood pressure. It can be fatal if consumed in a large amount.

22

"MCGARBAGE, MCCANCER" THE LARGEST INFECTION

"Eat McDonalds and Become a Big Mac"

- One in four people in America visit a fast food restaurant every day
- Fast food restaurants distribute lots of toys to children
- Contribute to obesity and disease
- Approximately 50 million people eat at McDonald's everyday

High Calories in Fast Food Restaurants

- White Castle - 20 chicken rings, **1,760 calories**
- Burger King - Ultimate breakfast platter, **1,450 calories**
- McDonald's - Big breakfast w/ syrup and margarine, **1,350 calories**
- KFC - 10-piece original recipe chicken bites, **1,300 calories**
- Wendy's - Hot 'N Juicy 3/4 lb. triple w/ cheese, **1,120 calories**
- Panera Bread - Steak and white cheddar on baguette, **980 calories**
- Taco Bell - Volcanic nachos, **970 calories**
- Dunkin' Donuts - Frozen mocha coffee coolatta, **730 calories**
- Subway - Mega melt on flatbread with egg, **660 calories**
- Pizza Hut - 14-inch large meat lover's pan pizza, **470 calories**
- Burger King Triple Whopper — **1,020 calories**
- Quizno's large Veggie Deluxe sandwich - **1,060 calories**

༈ Cinnabon's Caramel Pecanbon - **1,080 calories**
༈ Mountain Dew Baja Blast at Taco Bell XL **- 1,134 calories**

"Holy Kleenex Batman, it was right under our noses and we blew it! – Robin!"

You blew it alright, if you continue on the fast food track. Just looking at the above calories should be a major deterrent to never go to a fast food restaurant. And if you think you can get away with just a drink, check out the whopping calorie drinks at Dunkin Donuts and Taco Bell. Don't be fooled, there are hidden calories and junk at almost all fast food restaurants. Fast food can increase the risk of hardening and narrowing of the arteries, heart disease and stroke due to the types of ingredients it contains and the high quantities that people consume.

Let's talk junk in fast food

Trans-fats - saturated trans-fat add hydrogen to liquid vegetable oils. Trans-fats, also known as partially hydrogenated oils, raise your unhealthy cholesterol levels, leading to fatty plaques and hardening of the arteries.

Sugar - is included in all beverages such as fruit juice, milkshakes, and sodas. High sugar consumption can lead to obesity and an increase in Type 2 diabetes.

Sodium – Commercial processing and preparation make fast foods high in sodium. French Fries add 335mg before they've been sprinkled with salt, two pancakes with syrup has 1,104mg of sodium, and a roast beef sandwich contains 792mg of sodium. The average consumption of sodium for a healthy person is 2300mg. I recommend using pink salt from Premier and don't consume the unhealthy white salt used in most restaurants.

Calories - Weight gain and obesity. When eating at a fast food restaurant we usually eat too many calories all at one time. High fat and sugar content can lead to cardiovascular disease.

Chipotle is a fast food restaurant I recommend, and I promise I don't own stock in their company. Many of their items are organic and they offer a salad that can be ordered with beans. If you pass on the cheese, you can keep it healthy and lower in calories, although the cheese is actually organic!

Cancer is Very Misunderstood

It is a medical fact that every person has millions of cancer cells in their body at all times in their life. It takes many years, or even decades, for these so-called "malignant" tumors to grow. These millions of cancer cells remain undetectable through standard tests. However, they show up as tumors once they have multiplied to several billion. The body turns over 30 billion cells each day, and approximately 1% become damaged and turn cancerous. The immune system is programmed to detect these cancer cells and sends in a task force to repair the damage. White blood cells kill germs and infections. Red blood cells carry oxygen from the lungs to other cells. Cells turn cancerous when they lack oxygen, glucose and are nutrient deprived. But when the army gets weak, and when our immune system cannot repair the damage, we start losing the war.

As long as the causes of tumor growth remain intact, meaning people continue to increase toxicity in their body, cancer will redevelop in another area. If a doctor removes a tumor and a person does not make changes, this will increase the chances cancer will grow to a large enough size that it can be detected somewhere else in the body. "Cancer is not a disease; in fact all diseases are a final and most desperate attempt to get your attention to heal your body." Healing is accepting, allowing and supporting the body, not fighting and resisting. Modern procedures to fight cancer are chemotherapy and radiation which does not fight disease; it fights the body. If a car breaks down you want to repair the cause of the malfunction, not put a band aid on it. Disease means something is wrong with our engine. If your car is lacking oil, you put oil to help it to run. When our bodies are sick we need to put the right nutrients in to give us the fuel to run efficiently.

Carbohydrates fuel cancer cells. Cancer cells use glucose blood sugar as their "food." Carbs suppress the immune system, making a person more susceptible to cancer.

In a recent Canadian study, 70 percent of mice on a high-carb western-like diet developed tumors, while only 30 percent of the low-carb group grew tumors. Here are the details of their diets. The high-carb mice consumed a diet of 55 percent carbs, 23 percent protein, and 22 percent fat, and

70 percent developed tumors. The low-carb group ate a diet of 15 percent carbs, 25 percent fat, and 60 percent protein and only 30 percent developed tumors.

How Diet Effects Cancer

"Normal cells can function using energy from both fat and sugar [carbohydrates]," says study coauthor Gerald Krystal, Ph.D., professor at the University of British Columbia. "But cancer cells depend more heavily on glycolysis, a process that breaks down only sugar, for energy."

Researchers have shown that human cancer cells feast on your blood sugar after a high carb meal and multiply rapidly. So the opposite is true to eliminate carbs and junk from your diet so that the cancer cells will not have anything to feast on and will die.

Otto H. Warburg from 1931 and 1944 theorizes that the prime cause of cancer is the replacement of the respiration of oxygen in normal body cells by a fermentation of sugar. All normal body cells meet their energy needs by respiration of oxygen, whereas cancer cells meet their energy needs in great part by fermentation. All normal body cells are thus obligate aerobes, whereas all cancer cells are partial anaerobes. From the standpoint of the physics and chemistry of life this difference between normal and cancer cells is so great that one can scarcely picture a greater difference. Oxygen gas, the donor of energy in plants and animals is dethroned in the cancer cells and replaced by an energy yielding reaction of the lowest living forms, namely, a fermentation of glucose.

Otto Warburg won the Nobel Prize in 1932 for proving that cancer needs an anaerobic (oxygen-poor) environment in order to thrive. As the body's pH drops, less and less oxygen is available to tissues. So I would hypothesize that cancer will grow much easier in an unhealthy acidic body.

Worldwide research in the last 10 years points to chronic infection as the underlying driving force behind cancer. It is well known that long term inflammation, 7 or 8 years is highly correlated to the onset of cancer. In 1974, Seymour Halpern at Cornell University showed that you cannot get an infection unless you are first nutrient deficient.

In the book **The China Study,** by T Colin Campbell, Professor Emeritus of Nutritional Biochemistry at Cornell University, and his son Thomas M. Campbell II present information that is a definite challenge to the dairy and beef industries by revealing how dangerous these products are to human health.

Campbell is a professor who has spent 40 years in nutrition research and was the leader of the China Study, which was a combined study from Cornell University, Oxford University, and the Chinese Academy of Preventive Medicine.

This study involved 65 counties in 24 different provinces of China. The study looked at death rates from cancer and chronic diseases from 1973 -75. They took blood work from 100 people in each country. The study compared affluent areas where people consumed more meat and dairy products which had a higher rate of cancers of breast, prostate and bowel, diabetes and heart disease to poverty areas where they did not consume meat proteins and were less likely to die from those diseases. The authors concluded that those living in rural communities and consuming mostly plant protein had fewer chronic diseases that those who lived in communities where more animal protein was available.

In previous experiments, with rats, Campbell was able to show that with a diet of 20% casein (a milk protein) rats developed carcinogenic tumors. Switching the rats to a plant-based diet resulted in a decrease in tumor growth. Switching back to the casein diet brought renewed tumor growth. He was able to conclude that animal-based foods increased tumors while plant-based foods decreased the development of tumors.

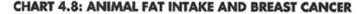

CHART 4.8: ANIMAL FAT INTAKE AND BREAST CANCER

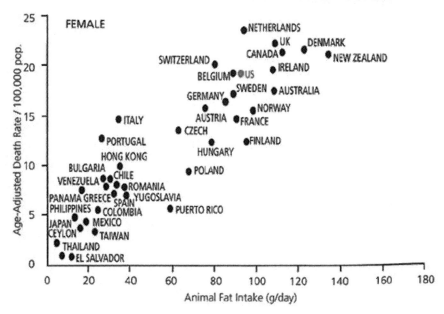

Cancer does not kill a person afflicted with it! There is nothing in a cancer cell that has the ability to kill anything. Curing cancer has little to do with getting rid of a cluster of cancer cells. Modern treatment with chemotherapy and radiation poisons or burns many cancer cells. However, they also destroy healthy cells in the bone marrow, gastrointestinal tract, liver, kidneys, heart, lungs, etc., which often leads to permanent irreparable damage of entire organs and systems in the body. A real cure of cancer does not occur by destroying other vital parts of the body. The sad truth is that many people do not die from cancer they die from the effects of what chemo and radiation has done to their bodies; the wasting away of cell tissue due to being deprived of nutrients. If you observe the withering leaves in the fall, it is important to notice that the leaves are dehydrated, meaning they are lacking nourishment. This is the same process to describe how disease processes in the human body. If we don't have proper nourishment, we ourselves will become sick and die.

What kills a cancer patient is not the tumor, but the numerous reasons behind cell mutation and tumor growth!

Cancer is a survival mechanism, not a disease. It is the final and most desperate survival mechanism the body has at its disposal. It only takes control of the body when all other measures of self-preservation have failed. To truly heal cancer and what it represents in a person's life we must come to the understanding that the reason the body allows some of its cells to grow in abnormal ways is in its best interest and not an indication that it is about to destroy itself. Cancer is a healing attempt by the body for the body. Blocking this healing attempt can destroy the body. Supporting the body in its healing efforts can save it.

Andreas Moritz's book, Cancer is not a Disease - It's a Survival Mechanism, explains the root causes of cancer and how to eliminate them for good. If you have cancer, please read this book. It is the most amazing book I have ever read.

23

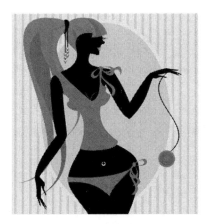

"WHAT COMES DOWN, WILL GO UP" YOYO DIETING

Yo-yo dieting is the ups and downs, and having to deal with the frustrations of on again off again dieting. Many people can lose weight, but then go off their diets, gain the weight back and just can't seem to keep it off. This can be very confusing for your metabolism with this repeat dieting, where the body starts to hold on to every calorie you eat. I have tried every diet there is, the latest and greatest, each an attempt to lose the weight...again. For a while I would lose weight because I would pick a different type of diet, like, Weight Watcher's to the cabbage soup diet. Since it was a different type of diet, it would boost my metabolism. After getting used to that diet, my weight loss would come to a halt...yet again.

When you are in line at the supermarket do you look over at the celebrities on the front pages of the magazines? It's no wonder that we try to starve ourselves to look like what we think we should. Most of us have no idea what a lot of money can buy such as: a personal chief and personal trainer that help rich celebrities stay in shape. Also, many of the photos are photo shopped, making the women look smaller than they are. These distorted images make us want to be something that is not even real....Fake!

Many of us, including me, have made the mistake of eating too little, restricting calories, which will prevent our bodies from burning fat storage efficiently. Then the body starts to hold on to the food and fat thinking it is in starvation mode. The body is so intelligent that when it does not have enough calories it makes the most of the calories it has, meaning it slows down the metabolism. The body actually protects the fat and to keep the body functioning it uses muscle to provide the calories. Your body is designed to store fat. Fat is your principal energy store and your body does not want to deplete it unless it absolutely has to. So with too few calories, you burn more muscle each time, becoming fattier, and slowing your metabolism. If we build up more muscle this means a higher metabolism and more fat burn. So you have gained nothing by eating too little, in fact you lose out by not enjoying and nourish yourself and becoming fatter.

How many wives have started a diet with their husbands and they lose twice as much as you do. Men have a much higher muscle mass than women so they will most likely always be the winners in weight loss. Not Fair! It has been charted that for every 10 pounds of muscle one can burn an extra 500 calories without doing anything. Now that makes sense when you see lean muscular people and they can eat much more than you and not gain weight. You know the person that is thin as a rail and goes back for three servings on the buffet! So the final answer is: Strength training, weight lifting. Get out of your rut and hit the gym. Build up your muscle mass, especially if you have been a yoyo'er; since you know now that every time you put the weight back on you gained fat. Muscle tissue is responsible for most of the calories that you burn each day, so your body needs good healthy protein to feed your muscle.

Forget crash dieting or any thoughts of rapid weight loss.

The safe rate at which you can lose weight is 1-2lbs a week. That doesn't sound a lot but equates to 52-104lbs a year!

1. **Eat a good source of protein to restore your metabolism.**
   Protein stimulates your fat burning metabolism as your body produces glucagon - your fat burning hormone - when you eat foods that contain

protein. Remember that muscle is made of protein. When working out, especially weightlifting, rev up your protein intake. Make sure to eat good quality fish, nuts, seeds, lean organic meats, organic eggs, and vegetables (which also contain protein). Limit or do not use dairy for your protein supply. Use Premiers Trim Body Whey; it is fabulous.

2. **Eat every 3-4 hours**
Regular eating helps to maintain balanced blood sugar levels, so you won't feel hungry and your body gets the energy it needs to function effectively. I have always been a grazer, eating 6 small meals a day. Remember to add lots of fruits and vegetable to help keep you full and satisfied.

3. **Take supplements to keep your thyroid healthy**
Yo-yo dieting can interfere with the functioning of your thyroid gland, which secretes thyroxine. Thyroxine plays an important role in your metabolism. Eat foods rich in iodine, such as seaweed, which can be found in more and more supermarkets and japanese salads, for instance. Take Premiers supplements Green Tea, Premier Greens (blue green algae and spirulina) and Xenostat to help give the proper nutrients to help keep the thyroid functioning. Do not use table salt; it is an unhealthy way to get iodine since salt is a chemical.

4. **Exercise regularly**

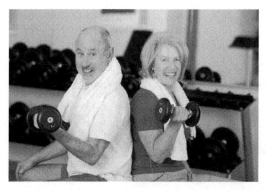

You definitely need to exercise. Remember you can start with walking and yoga. Exercise burns fat and weight lifting builds muscle. It is as simple as that. You need to raise your metabolism to burn more calories. Eventually you will need to start lifting weights. It does not mean extremely heavy weights, you can start very light. You need to build muscle and reduce fat to rev up the furnace in your body to burn more fat. This will help tremendously to keep the fat off, as you may be able to consume more food without gaining weight.

For more inspiration, consider some of the key findings from more than 10,000 people who have lost at least 30 pounds and kept it off for at least a year. They shared their strategies with the National Weight Control Registry, which posted them on its website:

- 78% eat <u>breakfast</u> every day.
- 75% weigh themselves at least once a week.
- 62% watch less than 10 hours of TV per week.
- 90% <u>exercise</u>, on average, about 1 hour per day.

"The process of converting consumed products into energy is your metabolism. Your body is constantly burning calories to repair cells, help you breathe, circulate blood and adjust hormones. Your size, age, body composition and gender affect this resting level of your metabolism. Activity also affects your metabolism--the more you move, the more energy your body needs and your metabolism revs in response. Finally, digestion accounts for about 10 percent of your metabolic burn, according to MayoClinic.com."

Muscle burns a lot more calories than fat so when we lose muscle, our metabolic rate drops and we burn fewer calories. When you lose weight quickly on an extreme diet, you are losing lean muscle along with fat. If you do not exercise during your diet, this magnifies the fat gain. If you are a yo-yoer, you are will most likely regaining mostly fat only, according to Dr. Michael Roizen and Dr. Mehmet Oz in "You, On A Diet."

How many Calories should you eat?

So here is the million dollar question. I believe that women should never dip below 1200 calories a day and men no lower than 1800. I don't really believe that it is about the calories; it is about the type of foods you eat. As for calories for women, I feel that women should not go below 1400 if they exercise every day, more if it is an exerting exercise.

If you are really sick then I suggest mostly a raw diet, lots of fresh raw juicing and a good source of protein in a smoothie using Premiers Lean Body Whey. I know this can be hard, and many of you already have allergies, autoimmune diseases and inflammation in your body. I recommend you get tested with QRA as soon as possible.

Here is my daily regime

7:30 am hot green tea (nothing else in it)

8:30am Start on my homemade Gatorade I call Cherryade (recipe to follow)

11:00am Homemade raw juice or smoothie (add trim body whey to both)

12:00pm Continue drinking Cherryade and raw nuts, Kombucha (probiotic drink)

1:00pm Salad (lots of raw veggies with fermented cabbage on top) and fruit

2:00pm Raw Nuts, Guacamole w/ seed crackers, hummus

3:00pm Fruits

5:00pm Smoothie with Trim Body Whey, scrambled eggs, fish,

pinto beans, sweet potato or brown rice

7:00pm Dark Chocolate 70 percent minimum, hot tea

Cherryade Energy Drink

Max B-ND™ is a probiotic-cultured B vitamins 1 teaspoon

Fresh Cherry Elixade Use 1 ounce

1/2 to 1 teaspoon pink salt

28 ounces of Water

This book is filled with many healthy food choices, mostly recommending consuming as much raw fruits and vegetables as possible. It doesn't mean that I don't cheat; I am human....I think! We will all have days when we falter, so keep a positive attitude and get right back to a healthy diet. "Healthy diet, healthy body."

24

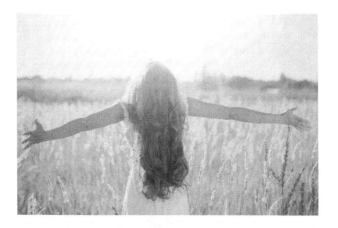

"LET THE SUN SHINE IN, THE SUN SHINE IN"
SUNLIGHT AND SUNBATHING

The sun is responsible for all life on earth. The sun does not cause cancer. If so, why didn't farmers thirty years ago get cancer? They were out in the sun all day. Could it be something that has changed over the years like crappy food? There are researches that theorize that the answer is the depressed immune function and toxicity. That would make more sense.

Plants grow outside in the sun all day. If they do not have enough nutrients in the soil and water they will die. The same is true for us; we need the proper nutrients to survive and thrive. We need internal protections instead of toxic sunscreens. If you work in the sun all day it is recommended to wear a long sleeve shirt and hat to protect yourself. Many of us are inside all day. Having the right nutrition is key; so if you are looking to get healthier, take your nutrients and vitamins and get your natural vitamin D outside.

Sunlight has been known to help lower blood sugar. Sunlight helps to store the sugar as glycogen in the liver, muscles and cells for later use. Being in the sun also helps stimulate the capillaries and bring blood to the surface.

Sunlight has been known to strengthen digestion and improve the eyesight. It is recommended to not wear sunglasses and to use Gods sunglasses, blinking. If you can't give up the sunglasses, at least let your eyes take in about ten minutes of sun a day. That should be easy for you as you take your ten minute walk outside.

The sun has also been given credit for helping with hormone balance and we all know it helps with depression and well-being. My eighty year old mother in law has been depressed for years. We went to see her in the nursing home and noticed she was very dark. We almost did not recognize her. She told us she was spending hours sun bathing each day. What we did notice, is that she was the happiest and healthiest we had seen her in a long time.

Note: If you burn easy or if you are just starting to sun bath, you must use common sense and take it easy. *"An hour of sun can take some dis-ease away."*

"Sacrifice what you are now, for what you can become tomorrow."

There is no ending, just beginnings; you are closing a door to unhealthy habits and opening a window of opportunities to change your life forever. Knowledge has to be learned. To earn knowledge you must have an honest desire to achieve it. To heal you must be willing to go to any lengths by staying motivated, visualizing, and believing in yourself. "A dream is a wish your heart makes." So make your dream come true. Make that change and bring health and joy back into your life. This book offers everything you need to regain your health. There are so many reasons that explain why we stops being able to lose weight. You have learned it can be from poor diet, poor digestion, genetics, hormone imbalance, inflammation, infections, starvation diets, emotional and physical stress, adrenal fatigue, and toxic teeth. Most of you are going to have a combination of issues, so you will need to start cleaning up your life one day at a time.

I hope you will take away the knowledge in this book and understand how dangerous and poisonous the foods and drinks are in today's world. Many of you already have food sensitivities and allergies to foods, which is the start of a weakened immune system and inflammation in the body. It is a final attempt or warning sign from your body begging you to feed it nutritious food. Many of you are already so sick you will have to detox your body from a lifetime of abuse because the sickness is infiltrated into your organs, tissue and fat. "Food for thought" change your ways or you will be sick and stay sick. There is no medical procedure/medication that will change this. "Feed a body nutrients, and starve the toxins."

There is no need to worry about the amount of calories you consume. This does not mean consuming a lot of toxic junk food, it means eating healthy real, live food. Don't be tricked into eating the fake, processed diet food, with the low calories, high carb and high sugar ingredients. For those of you who are just starting a diet, you will lose weight. For those of you who have been chronic dieters the toxins will start adding up and you will get to the point where you cannot lose weight. Make sure to eat from the list below as often as possible.

Lisa's food pyramid in this order:

Veggie/Fruit Group - Organic Vegetables, organic fruits, raw organic homemade juice

Protein Group - Wild Caught Fish, organic meats, organic free roaming eggs, raw nuts and seeds, avocado and hummus.

Fat Group - Raw nuts and seeds, avocado, EFA oils, DHA oil

Carbohydrates - Sweet Potatoes, organic brown rice, purple potatoes

Make sure to keep you protein high to help boost your immune system and metabolic rate. Balance your meals and rotate your foods to help steady blood sugar and to burn stored fat. Drink plenty of water, if you don't you will be "treading on thin ice" and toxic buildup will have no outlet. Eat 6 small meals a day to keep your energy up and make sure you are consuming fiber(fruits and vegetables) all day to help keep you full, to push food through your digestive track and fill your body with natural antioxidants, vitamins and nutrients. Try some dehydrated snacks such as raw crackers or chewy dried fruits.

Try to focus on a positive attitude, especially if you are not losing weight right away. If your body is ill, you will need to be patient, as your body will take time to heal before you can lose weight. If you start an exercise program remember that muscle weighs more than fat, so don't be obsessed with the scales.

Be well. All questions call be directed to WhycantIloseweight@yahoo.com.

BIBLIOGRAPHY

U.S. Food and Drug Administration FDA. (2012, May). "Keep Listeria Out of Your Kitchen" http://www.fda.gov/forconsumers/consumerupdates/ucm274114.htm

U.S. Food and Drug Administration FDA. (2014, August). Import Alert: 16-131. http://www.accessdata.fda.gov/cms_ia/importalert_33.html

Environmental Protection Act EPA. (2010, June). Mold-Indoor Community Health Risk.
http://www.epa.gov/osp/tribes/NatForum10/ntsf10_3t_Munoz.pdf

Marks Daily Apple. (2014, June) "The Lowdown on Lectins" http://www.marksdailyapple.com/lectins/#ixzz3EwBtZGfG

Proceedings of the National Academy of Sciences of the United States of America. (2009). http://en.wikipedia.org/wiki/Proceedings_of_the_National_Academy_of_Sciences_of_the_United_States_of_America

Good Fats 101. . (2013, November). "Good Fats vs Bad Fats" http://www.goodfats101.com/fats-101/good-vs-bad/#sthash.O51wz0Vp.dpuf

Centers for Disease Control and Prevention. "Carbohydrates. http://www.cdc.gov/nutrition/everyone/basics/carbs.html

Damy Health (2009-2014) "Processed Foods: Eliminate White Sugar and White Flour" http://www.damyhealth.com/processed-foods-white-sugar-white-flour/

U.S. Food and Drug Administration FDA (2013, September). Arsenic in Rice and Rice. Productshttp://www.fda.gov/food/foodborneillnesscontaminants/metals/ucm319870.htm

Central for Disease and Control Prevention (2012, October). "Consumption of Diet Drinks in the United States, 2009–2010". http://www.cdc.gov/nchs/data/databriefs/db109.htm

Center for Disease and Control Prevention. (2011, August) "Consumption of Sugar Drinks in the United States, 2005–2008". http://www.cdc.gov/nchs/data/databriefs/db71.htm

Center for Disease and Control Prevention. (2014) "Estimates of Diabetes and Its Burden in the United States" http://www.cdc.gov/diabetes/pubs/statsreport14/national-diabetes-report-web.pdf

Homestead Style (2012, August). Nuts and Seeds Chart. http://homesteadstyle.com/nut-seed-nutritional-chart/

U.S. Food and Drug Administration FDA .(2013, August) "FDA Continues to Study BPA". http://www.fda.gov/forconsumers/consumerupdates/ucm297954.htm

Susan E. Brown & Larry Trivieri, Jr., (2006) "The Acid-Alkaline Food Guide", SquareOne Publishers Garden City Park, NY,

The Prime Cause and Prevention of Cancer - Part 1, http://healingtools.tripod.com/primecause1.html/

Hormone Balancing Act Chart. prettystrongblog.blogspot.com

U.S. Food and Drug Administration (FDA). (2014, April). "Requirements for Specific New Drugs or Devices." http://www.accessdata.fda.gov/scripts/cdrh/cfdocs/cfcfr/cfrsearch.cfm?fr=310.545

Delicious Obsessions. (2012, April). "52 Uses for Coconut Oil" http://www.deliciousobsessions.com/2012/01/52-uses-for-coconut-oil-the-simple-the-strange-and-the-downright-odd/

Nature – Weekly International Journal of Science (2008, March) "Dynamics of fat cell turnover in humans," http://www.nature.com/nature/journal/v453/n7196/full/nature06902.html

Clarence and Carol Bass. (2014). "Exercise Activates Genes Regulating Fat and Muscle." http://www.cbass.com/controlgenes.htm

Red Orbit. (2005) "Genes May Influence Weight Gain in Adults" http://www.redorbit.com/news/health/122143/genes_may_influence_weight_gain_in_adults/#bUUScfqPDeLuGU4v.99

Diagnose Me.com (2014, October). "Mercury Toxicity (Amalgam Illness)." http://www.diagnose-me.com/symptoms-of/mercury-toxicity-amalgam-illness.html

U.S. Food and Drug Administration (FDA). (2014, June) "About Dental Amalgam Fillings" http://www.fda.gov/medicaldevices/productsandmedicalprocedures/dentalproducts/dentalamalgam/ucm171094.htm#4

U.S. Food and Drug Administration (FDA). (2014, July). "FDA Update/Review of Potential Adverse Health Risks Associated with Exposure to Mercury in Dental Amalgam." http://www.fda.gov/medicaldevices/productsandmedicalprocedures/dentalproducts/dentalamalgam/ucm171117.htm

Trivieri, Larry, and John W. Anderson. Alternative Medicine: The Definitive Guide. Second ed. Celestial Arts, 2002. http://www.naturalnews.com/045704_dental_problems_root_canals_oil_pulling.html?utm_content=buffer8554a&utm_medium=social&utm_source=facebook.com&utm_campaign=buffer#ixzz3I3tfXobN

Frederick W. Kutz, Patricia H. Wood, David P. Bottimore. (1991), "Organochlorine Pesticides and Polychlorinated Biphenyls in Human Adipose Tissue" http://link.springer.com/chapter/10.1007%2F978-1-4612-3080-9_1

Center for Emerging Issues, Centers for Epidemiology and Animal Health Animal and Plant Health Inspection Service, USDA. "Dioxins in the Food

Chain:Background." http://www.aphis.usda.gov/animal_health/emergingissues/downloads/dioxins.pdf

The Corisol Connection. "Cortisol, Stress & Abdominal Fat"(2000). http://cortisol.com/cortisol-stress-abdominal-fat/#.VFjlNcmObxg

Walter J. Crinnion ND.(2000). "Environmental Medicine: Excerpts from Articles on Current Toxicity, Solvents, Pesticides and Heavy Metals." http://www.tldp.com/issue/210/environmen.htm

The Healthy Back Institute. (2008, July). "10 Foods That Naturally Relieve Pain and Inflammation." http://www.losethebackpain.com/blog/2008/07/24/10-foods-that-reduce-inflammation-and-pain-naturally/

Albers, S. (2009). *50 ways to Soothe Yourself without Food.* New Harbinger Publications.

Barnard, N.D. & Stepaniak, J. (2004). *Breaking the Food Seduction: The Hidden Reasons behind Food Cravings and 7 Steps to End Them*

Doreen Virtue. "Constant Craving" (2011, September) Hay House.com

Neal D. Barnard, Joanne Stepaniak. (2004, September). Breaking the Food Seduction: The Hidden Reasons Behind Food Cravings---And 7 Steps to End Them Naturally Paperback

Francis Marion Pottenger Jr. (1995, June). "Pottenger's Cats: A Study in Nutrition"

The Washington Times Communities. (2011, March) "Drugging America: The drug industry exposed." http://communities.washingtontimes.com/ neighborhood/omkara/2011/mar/27/dark-secrets-drug-industry-exposed/

Science Daily. (2008, January). "Big Pharma Spends More On Advertising Than Research And Development, Study Finds". http://www.sciencedaily. com/releases/2008/01/080105140107.htm

Non GMO Project. (2014) The "Non-GMO Project Verified" Seal. http:// www.nongmoproject.org/learn-more/understanding-our-seal/

Life Sources, Inc. (1998 April) "The 12 most Dangerous Prescription Drugs." http://www.life-sources.com/pages/The-12-most-Dangerous-Prescription-Drugs....html

U.S. Food and Drug Administration (FDA). (2007, July) "How FDA Regulates Seafood." http://www.fda.gov/downloads/forconsumers/consumerupdates/ ucm106813.pdf

U.S. Food and Drug Administration (FDA). (2013, December) "Phasing Out Certain Antibiotic Use in Farm Animals." http://www.fda.gov/forconsumers/ consumerupdates/ucm378100.htm

U.S. Food and Drug Administration (FDA). "Steroid Hormone Implants Used for Growth in Food-Producing Animals." http://www.fda.gov/ animalveterinary/safetyhealth/productsafetyinformation/ucm055436.htm

Ganmaa Davaasambuu, Harvard University Gazette (2006, December). "Hormones in Milk Can Be Dangerous." http://news.harvard.edu/ gazette/2006/12.07/11-dairy.html

U.S. Food and Drug Administration (FDA. (2013, September)

"Questions & Answers: Arsenic in Rice and Rice Products" http://www.fda.gov/Food/FoodborneIllnessContaminants/Metals/ucm319948.htm

Health Guidance. Adam Brookover. "Dangers of Food Additives and Preservatives." http://www.healthguidance.org/entry/9987/1/Dangers-of-Food-Additives-and-Preservatives.html

Ashley Lutz and Jennifer Welsh Business Insider. (2013, May) "17 Of The Highest-Calorie Chain Restaurant Items" http://www.businessinsider.com/17-highest-calorie-chain-restaurant-items-2013-5?op=1#ixzz3HMCbL6ZT

Andreas Moritz. (2008, August) "Cancer Is Not a Disease - It's a Survival Mechanism."

Hodnett-AP - Hormones and Endocrine System Chart. Rita Zeng. hodnett-ap.wikispaces.com

Thomas Campbell and T. Colin Campbell. "The China Study: The Most Comprehensive Study of Nutrition Ever Conducted And the Startling Implications for Diet, Weight Loss, And Long-term Health." (2006, May)

Prmom Life. (2011). "Specifics About Each Of The Five Metals" http://www.promolife.com/cart/health-articles/detox-articles/heavy-metals-bodys-time-bomb

LiveStrong.com. Clay McNight (2014, February). "Three Main Dangers of Dieting". http://www.livestrong.com/article/352609-three-main-dangers-of-dieting/

Dr. Myatte The Wellness Club. (2014). "10 Dangers of Carbohydrates." http://www.drmyattswellnessclub.com/DangersOfCarbohydrates.htm

U.S. Food and Drug Administration (FDA). (2014, October). "Steroid Hormone Implants Used for Growth in Food-Producing Animals" http://www.fda.gov/AnimalVeterinary/SafetyHealth/ProductSafetyInformation/ucm055436.htm

WebMed. "What Are Weight Cycling and Yo-Yo Dieting?" http://www.webmd.com/diet/weight-cycling

Huff Post. "Fat Genes' Determine Obesity, UCLA Study Says, In Addition To Diet And Exercise." (2014, February). http://www.huffingtonpost.com/2013/01/10/fat-genes-obesity-ucla-study-diet-exercise_n_2450108.html

Naturally. St. Martin's Griffin.Virtue, D. (2011). "Constant Craving: What Your Food Cravings Mean and How to Overcome Them." Hay House.

[Johnson, J.A. and Bootman,, J. L. "Drug-Related Morbidity and Mortality: A Cost-of-Illness Model." *Archives of Internal Medicine*, 1995; 155:1949-1956.]

New England Journal of Medicine ["Emergency Hospitalizations for Adverse Drug Events in Older Americans"], http://www.nejm.org/search?q=emergency+hospitalizations+for+adverse+drug+events+in+older+americans&asug=emergency+h

Annemarie Colbin, Ph.D. (1997) "Cholesterol – Is it really so bad?" http://www.foodandhealing.com/articles/article-cholesterol.htm

Non GMO Project. (2014), What is GMO? Agricultural Crops That Have a Risk of Being GMO. http://www.nongmoproject.org/learn-more/what-is-gmo/

Scientific Reports. (2013, January). "High arsenic in rice is associated with elevated genotoxic effects in humans." http://www.nature.com/srep/2013/130722/srep02195/full/srep02195.html. Detoxification During Weight Loss

Byron J. Richards. (2013, March), "Detoxification During Detox.". http://www.
wellnessresources.com/weight_tips/articles/detoxification_during_weight_loss/.

William Gamonski. "Foods that Reduce Cortisol Levels." http://www.
wellnessresources.com/weight_tips/articles/detoxification_during_weight_loss/.

AltMed, "Chiropractic Care for Stress." http://altmd.com/Articles/Chiropractic-
Care-for-Stress

Laura Gee. "How to Lose Weight by Eating Raw Foods." http://www.ehow.
com/how_5515785_lose-weight-eating-raw-foods.html

Made in the USA
Charleston, SC
18 November 2015